Eat Healthy...

Most of the Time!

Enjoy All God's Best!

Drew Williams

By

Drew Williams

All scripture quotations are taken from the New King James Version of the Bible unless otherwise noted.
The New King James Version / Thomas Nelson Publishers.
Nashville : Thomas Nelson, Inc., Copyright © 1982.

ISBN 0-9779017-0-X

1. Bible. English.

OPEN WATER, INC.
Publisher
3088 Grand Blanc Road
Grand Blanc, MI 48439
Visit our website at: www.openwaterpublishing.com

Dedication

To my wife, Mary, and our four lovely and
precious daughters; may you always live for Jesus.
It is my joy to love and serve you all.

Acknowledgements

Thanks to my wife for her tireless efforts to make things better, including this book. She helps me strive for excellence while encouraging me when I don't achieve it.

Thanks to my friends, Pastor Nicholas and Yvonne Mihailoff, for your encouragement and example, and for reading the manuscript.

Thanks to all my running friends for insights you may not even have known you were sharing. You are too numerous to name but I appreciate you all.

Thanks to Mike Hetfield of Dickinson Press for working with me through the process.

Last but not least, thanks to Susan Harring, who proved over and over how good it is to have someone help you who knows what the heck they're doing.

Table of Contents

Introduction

This just in, "The latest study reveals that eating may kill you. Stop eating!"

Oh, wait, not eating will definitely kill you. What are you to do?

Confused by all the studies, reports and diet offerings? There is good news. First, food is not your enemy. Food is fuel. It is necessary to sustain us. Food alone does not make us fat, nor does it make us sick or healthy. Food, like money, is a tool. We can use it properly or we can misuse it.

Of course, we can also enjoy it. Many a person who is skilled with certain tools will report that they *enjoy* their tools. Enjoyment is a godly thing as long as it doesn't turn into obsession and misuse.

Meanwhile, we have a multi-billion dollar industry all wrapped up around our dietary habits with both the world and the church chiming in on what we should or should not eat.

I want you to eat. I want you to eat enough food to keep from being hungry. I want you to be the weight that you and God agree you should be. I want you to be healthy and enjoy life to the fullest. I believe you can do all of these without over concentrating on your diet (or your budget, but that's another story).

That's not to say that I believe you can or should eat indiscriminately. A responsible lifestyle is one wherein we reflect the character of God and there is definitely some responsibility that goes along with our diets. The question is, who's responsible for your diet, and who should be telling you what to eat? Does anyone even know how every person in the world ought to eat? Who's to say what everyone should enjoy?

I will tell you now, before we get to the "meat" of the matter, I am not one who pretends to know what you like, or what specifically is best for you. I do not plan to suggest any recipes or my favorite foods because they may not be your favorites. What I do plan to tell you is the world has gone crazy over this stuff and the church, in many cases, is following along. There are so many diet plans available today that the choices are overwhelming. Enough, I say! Let liberty come! Not a liberty that leads to excess, rather a liberty that leads to peace as we put food in its proper place in our lives.

Join me now as we journey through the minefield of popular opinion and break through to the light of God's liberty.

Chapter One

Foundation

1 John 2:15 "Do not love the world or the things in the world. If anyone loves the world, the love of the Father is not in him. [16] For all that [is] in the world—the lust of the flesh, the lust of the eyes, and the pride of life—is not of the Father but is of the world. [17] And the world is passing away and the lust of it, but he who does the will of God abides forever."

Many Christians across the globe have joined in the trend of following science to the exclusion of the word of God. Believe it or not, this falls within the context of the verses above. I call this a trend for it is not a concept limited to our time, but it has been slowly creeping in over the centuries. The phenomenon of observing times, seasons and events and then drawing conclusions from them has ever been with us, however in our recent generations we have raised this to new levels.

It started with evolution for this era. Of course, at first believers fought against the alteration of centuries of understanding regarding the creation of the world, but they were fighting not only a secular view of creation but their own ignorance of science and an inability to clearly articulate any relationship between science and scripture. At the time many believers saw science as "anti-Christ" and thus appeared to be extremists, although well-intentioned. In the following decades believers attempted to "reconcile" creation with evolution. I recall one teaching that says, "Between Genesis 1:1 and 1:2 we don't know how many eons passed." The implication is that all the evolutionary things could have taken place between those two verses and then God started over.

Today the trend is toward Intelligent Design. Many scientists have recognized the harmony of science and scripture when viewing the creation of the universe, and many Bible scholars are discovering that same truth. Science has found more evidence for the creationist theory than for any concept of evolution beyond bullfrogs and butterflies.

This is indicative of the battle that wages, and has waged since before Moses went up the mountain. People generally don't want to seek to know God for themselves. That simply takes too much work, but they do want to believe what God says. Of course, when folks say they want to believe, what they really mean is, they want proof before they will believe. "Seeing is believing," has been a rallying cry of multitudes over generations.

This trend can be seen in so many elements of our society but none more prevalently than in the areas of diet, nutrition and exercise. On one hand you have the folks who, though well intentioned, would like to see us revert to the law. Scores of books have been written and sermons preached on the benefits of various foods or diets based on Old Testament teachings regarding these things. The problem we have is the majority of scriptural information provided is derived from scriptures pertaining to the law. While the law provided numerous *guidelines* regarding diet, and there now exists extensive science that explains what **might** happen when people eat differently than as directed in the Law, it is improper to conclude that we should follow Old Testament dietary guidelines. The reason is simple; the New Testament provides specific instructions to the contrary.

On the other hand, you have those who derive all their information from scientific studies. While these studies honestly reflect results they do so based on the premise that what is studied and demonstrated is truth. In reality these studies reveal facts, not truth. And the facts can easily vary from study to study depending greatly on the assumptions made by the study's designer. The studies also discount the attitude of the persons involved in the study.

We have all seen, heard or read about studies that contradict other studies. How do we then choose what to believe?

It is time balance and liberty were restored to all of you who have felt compelled to alter your diet in such a fashion as to be completely lacking in joy and full of bondage. If eating is a chore you have lost your joy and are full of bondage over dietary practices.

Paul wrote, "Stand fast therefore in the liberty by which Christ has made us free, and do not be entangled again with a yoke of bondage." (Galatians 5:1) Paul goes on to discuss in this chapter of Galatians that if you become circumcised Christ profits you nothing. His point is if you give yourself over to one aspect of the law, you are a debtor to keep the *whole* law (Galatians 5:3). This is a point which so many people are inclined to ignore as they attempt to bring natural thinking to spiritual living. 1 Corinthians 3:17 says, "Now the Lord is the Spirit; and where the Spirit of the Lord *is*, there *is* liberty." Remember, as believers we are called to live life from the spirit, not from the natural. In fact, Paul put it this way in Romans 8:5-8:

> "[5]For those who live according to the flesh set their minds on the things of the flesh, but those *who live* according to the Spirit, the things of the Spirit. [6]For to be carnally minded *is* death, but to be spiritually minded *is* life and peace. [7]Because the carnal mind *is* (an enemy of) God; for it is not subject to the law of God, nor indeed can (it) be. [8]So then, those who are in the flesh cannot please God."

In verse 2 of chapter 8 Paul wrote that, *"The law of the Spirit of Life in Christ Jesus has made me free from the law of sin and death."* Let's be perfectly clear regarding the "law of sin and death." First, it is very much like gravity, in that it is a universal constant. This law operates in the world we live in and affects all of us in varying degrees. Even the most spiritually minded believer is affected by this law in that their body is bound for death. There is only one way out of this life; death. We will all go by that route. There are no alternatives. *"And as it is appointed for men to die once, but after this the judgment."* (Hebrews 9:27) (Actually, there is one alternative and that is to be caught up with the Lord as Enoch and Elijah were, but that is a doctrine of some controversy and is appointed for the end of the age so we'll skip it here.)

Second, also like gravity, there are laws that can supersede this law. In this case "the law of the Spirit of Life in Christ Jesus." We can live free from the majority of the effects of the law of sin and death as we are transformed in our thinking. Even the world of psychology acknowledges that a change in thinking is a key to altering lifestyles, but they fall far short of the change that provides the liberty that God intends for us. Most changes only alter our involvement in the "law of sin and death" (see Ro. 8:5 & 6a above) rather than bringing us into the liberty God intends (Ro 8:6b above). If we simply alter our natural, or carnal, behaviors based solely on scientific, philosophical or legal information we are only moving from one carnal, or fleshly, behavior to another.

Before we go on let me explain "carnal". This word has often been related to "sinful". In fact, Webster's Dictionary offers these definitions: "1a: relating to or given to crude bodily pleasures and appetites. 1b: marked by sexuality."

While sinful behaviors are indeed carnal behaviors, it does not hold that all carnal behaviors are necessarily sinful. The word carnal as used in this chapter is from a Greek word; *sarkos*, and is often translated "flesh." One scholar provides this definition for *sarkos*: "This word describes *anything that is of the flesh, fleshly made, or fleshly conjured up or anything that is natural or of an unspiritual nature."* (Sparkling Gems from the Greek; p. 107, by Rick Renner; 2003) The English word carnal is from a Latin word, *carne*, which means primarily "meat," or the flesh stripped of the skin.

As we can see, any number of behaviors can fall under the heading of "carnal" as defined above. If we spend an excessive amount of our time and energy on our homes, cars, jobs, sports, diets or even our families, we can find ourselves operating in the "carnal." You can see from the list that I have presented topics about which the Bible is not silent (okay, maybe it is on cars). I did this to reveal a way of seeing the difference between how we think and how God thinks.

In particular our families are of great value to God and these relationships are dealt with in numerous verses of the Bible. If we are to have a strong family and raise godly children equipped to succeed in this life, we obviously need to spend some time thinking about our families. However, the time we spend in dealing with, planning for and thinking about our families needs to be that which is lived out according to God's instructions. "Husbands, love your wives, as Christ loved the church..." (Ep 5:25) "Wives reverence or respect your husbands." (Ep 5:33) "Children obey your parents in the Lord." (Ep 6:1) "You (parents), do not provoke your children to wrath." (Ep 6:4)

Just a few verses indicating God's instructions for families and yet we must also remember that Jesus said, "*If anyone comes to Me and does not hate his father and mother, wife and children, brothers and sisters, yes, and his own life also, he cannot be My disciple.*" That verse is strong in opposition to the many other instructions on the family; and a paradox. How is a man to love his wife and a woman to respect or reverence her husband when Jesus says to "hate" them? Matthew 10:37 provides some clarification for this truth.

> "He who loves father or mother more than Me is not worthy of Me. And he who loves son or daughter more than Me is not worthy of Me."

Jesus tells us that it is not a true "hate" of our family but a preference for our relationship with the Lord <u>above any other relationship</u>. Our love for God should be so great that the difference between it and our "love" for our family or friends would <u>seem</u> like hate by comparison. It is this kind of Love for God that permitted the early church to hold God in such high esteem even though their families may have been wiped out by the Roman government.

Before you close the book and toss it, let me temper my message with another truth. Jesus did say,

"Come to me, all you who labor and are heavy laden, and I will give you rest. Take my yoke upon you, and learn from me, for I am gentle and lowly in heart, and you will find rest for your souls. For my yoke is easy and my burden is light." (Matthew 11:28-30)

The Christian life is intended to be a life of peace and joy. In fact, the Bible says that the Kingdom of God is "righteousness, **peace and joy** in the Holy Spirit." (Romans 14:17) It also proclaims that the Fruit of the Spirit is "Love, joy peace,..." (Galatians 5:22) Jesus told us to ask for things in His name that our joy may be full (John 16:24). I am not advocating a Spartan life or existence. I am not advocating that we are hateful toward our families, nor am I saying we should not tell people of the goodness and love of God. In fact the Bible teaches that it is the very "goodness of God that brings sorrow to repentance." (2 Corinthians 7:10) God's love and goodness is a much more effective tool for inspiring repentance and discipleship than any preaching of wrath or a Spartan lifestyle. Very few people are flocking to monasteries to pursue a monk's life and truthfully God does not desire it to be so. How can we reach our world if we don't live among them?

Yet, Jesus did challenge those who claimed to believe with hard truths that were meant to identify their motives and to inspire them to make a genuine commitment. Without a genuine commitment, there is no real pursuit. If we don't pursue the things of God they will not accidentally fall in our laps. Even if they did we would not value them because they came too easily. Thomas Paine wrote concerning the Revolution in 1775, "What we obtain too cheap, we esteem too lightly." (The Crisis) Our salvation was not cheap. Nor will it be "easy" to see God's plan come to pass in our lives, but it is simple.

Neither salvation nor God's plan can be paid for in any way by our own efforts, and neither can God's love or favor. Salvation, God's love and His favor come only through faith which absolutely requires that we know and believe His word, first and foremost. Romans 10:17 says, *"So then faith comes by hearing, and hearing by the Word of God."* Hebrews 11.6 says, *"Without faith it is **impossible** to please God."* Not difficult, not challenging, impossible! That is not a man's creed or idea, it is God's. Reason against it, argue about it, and dispute it all you want. You are wrong. God is right. *"For what if some did not believe? Will their unbelief make the faithfulness of God without effect? Let God be true and every man a liar."* (Romans 3:3-4a)

When our reasoning, theories and ideas are contrary to scripture we are wrong and God is true. Psalm 100:5 says, *"The Lord is good, His mercy is everlasting and His truth endures to **all** generations."* Not to some generations, not many generations until man's intellect evolves, but to all generations. That means the truths God said millennia ago are still pertinent today. And that truth culminates in Jesus Christ. In John 14:6 Jesus said of Himself, *"I am the way, **the truth**, and the life, no man comes to* *the Father but by Me."* So what shall we believe? Are we to believe scientific theorists, religious or Christian theorists, nutritionists or other so called experts, or the Living Word?

I am committing my life to the Living Word.

Chapter Two

What is Everyone Saying?

Current Diet Theories in the World

Current diet theories have various names with Atkins, South Beach, and Weight Watchers being three of them. There is meal targeting with a target laid out and so-called best foods in the bulls eye with worst on the edges, (but sometimes the best of protein is the worst of carbs and fat, and so on). Once upon a time, and sometimes it resurges, there was the grapefruit diet.

There is a consistent onslaught of new dietary theories released on a regular basis. If you subscribe to any modern magazine you are inundated with "advice" and menu plans. If you go into any book store the section reserved for diet and nutrition takes a back seat to none. There are proponents of vitamins, proponents of minerals, sellers of supplements and untold numbers of cookbooks and recipes. In researching this chapter I entered "diet and nutrition" in one search engine and came up with 22,800,000 hits on one or both of those words. I reviewed the first 30 before entering the words, "christian diets." That search returned 605,000 hits.

On one site a list of topics regarding health and diet contained the following: Cholesterol; 10,000 steps; Vitamins; Low Carb; Organic Foods; Exercise; and Losing Weight. As I mentioned, mineral supplements are also becoming popular as our "soil is depleted from overuse" and vitamins and minerals are being lost from our food. At least that's the sales pitch for the mineral supplements. Of course, with all of these topics and the myriad more that exist, there are varying opinions and studies that prove or disprove the value of each topic.

Add to all this the government's New Food Pyramid, which you can access at www.mypyramid.gov. At this site you are able to enter in some information and customize the pyramid for your age, weight and body type. There is also a site for tracking how you're doing at www.mypyramidtracker.gov.

As with all the other theories there are detractors for the new government guidelines. Some comments were that it is too difficult to identify which foods are best for you, and it's too hard to determine how much you should be eating, i.e., servings or portion sizes. While that may be true I have found it to be true of many of the diets offered. For those that are very specific about portions I find that the foods they recommend are not foods that I like, or they are expensive to buy. In fact, USA Today had an article in 2005 that addressed this topic and found that in order for a person to follow the Atkins diet, or the South Beach diet, they were going to have to spend between 25 and 40 percent more than for a "conventional" diet (conventional meaning shopping by **price**, taste and by choice as most people do).

One problem with many of the diets that limit or eliminate one element; such as low carb, or low fat; is that people tend to be unable to remain on these diets for a long period of time. I realize that by the time you read this someone will respond, "I have," because they have. However, I personally do not know anyone who has been on the Atkins Diet, Weight Watchers, South Beach, Low Fat, Hyper Vitamin, and so on, who is on that diet or program today. I'm sure there are people out there who have maintained some variation of a diet, but that is not strict adherence. Why vary a diet if it is so good?

People go on diets because they desire to alter something about their lives that is unsatisfactory to them. There is a desire to want control as well as to "look and feel better." People go off diets because the diet is too restrictive, or they actually achieve a goal, or the discipline is too much. One man said, "People can't live on diets or budgets. They're not made that way. A diet may be necessary for a short time to bring something under control, a budget may be used to help get out of debt or save for something." (Nicholas Mihailoff; Pastor; University Chapel; Flint, Michigan.)

Living on diets or budgets all the time just produces tension, bondage and frustration. One family lived on a budget that was so restrictive they often ate only beans for dinner, because they bought them in bulk. The plan was to get out of debt and to take control of their finances in order to buy a house. However, once the goal was reached things did not change. Very little funds were allocated for the unexpected "kid expenses." The dad, the budget designer, continued to "control" the finances and the mom was cut out of the decisions, and money was reportedly still "very tight." That "budget" was a means of control by that father and not a means of achieving financial liberty as purported. Similar scenarios are acted out by those with eating disorders. Neither type of behavior is healthy.

A budget that is somewhat flexible and allows for the unexpected is far different than the types of "budgets" I am referring to. I agree that we should live within our means, a concept which lends itself to the later discussion of a fasted lifestyle. Don't quit on me yet.

Dieting, meaning following some specific plan for eating that is supposed to lead to weight loss, is a failure waiting to happen if the only method employed is a so-called diet plan. Your weight may be unsatisfactory, but if you don't alter your internal view of your body then no amount of dieting will achieve, long term, the desired result. You will quickly become unhappy with food choices or you will grow tired of the effort, and you will go off the diet. Many of the better programs (not diets) understand that people may grow tired of "the same old thing" or that if the effort is too great they will not continue and they have tried to address this in some fashion. Some have even realized that without a change in internal perception people will fail and they promote positive thinking as a means to that change.

While positive thinking is better than negative thinking, it is not the method given by God for changing your internal image. We need to understand what God said about who and what we are and think in His terms, not our own.

*   *   *

Current "Doctrine" in the Church

I use the title "the church" loosely because we are not one gloriously united body of believers. The church, as Jesus described it, is that collective membership united in the common bond of salvation or being born again. Many scholars refer to this as the Universal Church which is the "body of Christ." The Local Churches are smaller segments (molecules) of this body. The atoms of the body are every individual believer, for we are the church.

With our own bodies, individual parts do not all have the same function but are individual members that are connected together by our central nervous system and brain to share a common purpose, that of carrying our soul and spirit through this world. We interact with the world around us through our bodies using members that have different functions; i.e. our eyes, ears, noses, mouths and nerve endings. These are not equal to one another, but they are equivalent in that they provide important input to or from our minds.

In much the same way the local church interacts with the world around us in an effort to fulfill God's purposes in this world. Ideally every local church would have a common understanding of just what the overall purpose is and, using different methods, be striving to live out that purpose. Unfortunately it doesn't always work this way, and often the most vicious instigator of an attack against one local church will be another local church. My friends these things ought not to be so, to paraphrase James. (James 3:10)

The result is the vastly differing viewpoints on numerous doctrines including the topic at hand; Eating Healthy. While there are a number of programs available which reflect certain core aspects of my own "philosophy," (if you'll forgive my use of the word), there are many more which reflect a growing dependence on the same studies used in secular culture to direct us to specific diets, foods, minerals or vitamins. The difference between the secular programs and the Christian ones is usually a difference in references. While secular "gurus" tout various motivations, activities and hoped for results, Christian programs add biblical references to give credibility to their method.

Of course, the Bible, the inspired word of God, is to be our final directive, our primary authority for the way we live life and achieve victory. But any program that promotes either a greater focus on our own bodies or a greater focus on Old Testament Laws and practices is in contradiction to the grace and discipline that Jesus delivered to us.

As members of the body of Christ, we need to look to His word for our instruction but we need to do so according to our covenant. We are New Testament people and this must be our first and predominant resource.

Chapter Three

What's the Problem?

I believe this is a monumental question, not only for the topic of this book but for all of our efforts to live a life that is *"...worthy of the Lord, fully pleasing Him, being fruitful in every good work and increasing in the knowledge of God."* (Colossians 1.10)

The problem is with our thinking.

We look at (perceive) life from our natural mind. We attempt to take our definition of what will please the Lord and what are *good works* from our own perceptions, thoughts and ideas. Instead, we need to see what God says and go with that. We need to know His thoughts and His ways – and be willing to let those thoughts and ways become our thoughts and ways. We need to be transformed by the renewing of our minds to think His way.

(Romans 12:2) As I mentioned in the first chapter, when we have an opinion contrary to God's word we must realize that we are wrong! God said His ways are not our ways and His thoughts are not our thoughts. (Isaiah 55:8-9) But He does want us to know His thoughts and ways. Jesus came to "show (us) the Father." (John 14:6-11; Hebrews 1:3)

If a modern day media person or political liberal had been in the camp when God told Joshua to take Jericho and to utterly destroy it, allowing no one to survive (except Rahab and her family because she was a believer) they would have written editorials and gone on talk shows to denounce Joshua and question his ability to lead. They would have pushed for impeachment or a recall vote and made up bumper stickers that said things like, "Hate is Not a Family Value." They would have filibustered in congress in an attempt to tie up the whole thing in administrative procedures, and they would have sincerely believed they were "doing the right thing," and "showing compassion."

Yet, the God of the universe gave Joshua his instructions. (Of course, they would have asked questions such as, "How do you know it was God?" And they would have demanded that Joshua form a committee to study the situation.) Fortunately for Joshua he was only the earthly leader of a Theocracy, a kingdom in which God was the supreme ruler. He acted on God's word. Events at Jericho and throughout the history of Israel demonstrate that God knew exactly what He was talking about.

Example: God instructed the Israelites not to make any treaties with any of the people of the land because they would become a snare to Israel. One tribe devised a trap for Joshua and tricked him into believing they were from a far country. Joshua accepted their word <u>without</u> seeking God's counsel and made a treaty with them. Right after he did they crossed over some hills and found these people living right in their way. Joshua had made a mistake but God commanded they honor the treaty. He keeps His word, even when it is given by a man whom He has given authority to act for Him in the earth, (which is one reason it is completely wrong to try to blame God for bad things. God gave Adam dominion and authority, Adam gave it to Satan who had made himself God's mortal enemy).

Some would say that Joshua was not obligated to keep the covenant because those people lied and yet, God has an entirely different view. In order for God's word to be <u>true</u> all that God says must be true. When God directed that we are to "swear to (our) own hurt," He was providing insight into His own character and giving instruction regarding the value of covenants. God keeps His word. He does not keep part of His word. He does not keep His word only if it is convenient. He keeps His word. Joshua was the Prime Minister of a Theocracy and spoke for the King. The King gave Joshua that authority and was bound by Joshua's promise. However, the fruit of that agreement was precisely what God had said would happen if the children of Israel did not drive out <u>all</u> of the inhabitants of the land. He said they would become a snare to the people and lead them away to other (so-called) gods, and that is what happened. God is true!

(Be aware that when I say the Bible is true and God keeps all of His word, understand that the whole of the Bible is **truly recorded**, but not all the Bible is the recorded words spoken by God. What God keeps is the word He has declared. And He always keeps it in line with His Grace because Jesus fulfilled the Old Testament law. He didn't throw it out, He superseded it. Where there is a conflict between the Old and the New, the Old is superseded. Where the New is silent, the Old provides examples and principles, not rules and regulations.)

In an attempt to drive this point home a little more, let's take a look at Truth.

Webster's defines truth as: Sincerity in action, character or utterance; as the body of real things, events and facts; and as fidelity to an original or <u>to a standard,</u> (author's emphasis).

Fidelity is defined as: Accuracy in details or exactness.

Thus, God is sincere in action, character and speech and He is the creator of all of the real things (Genesis 1; John 1.3; Ep 3.9). He is exact in adhering to His standard. God is not schizophrenic. He does not promise one thing one day and something different the next. In fact, His word does not come back to Him without production but accomplishes what He says it will (Isaiah 55:11) because He watches over His word to perform it. (Jeremiah 28:6; 29:10; 33:14)

Of course, many will say that while they agree that God is able to keep His word, He doesn't always do exactly what we think He's going to do. "I prayed for my uncle (sister, brother, mother, father, friend) to be healed and they weren't." "I asked

God to get rid of my boss, who's a real jerk, and He didn't, I guess it's just my cross to bear." "I prayed for God to give me money to pay my bills and all I got were job offers."

I agree that we don't always get what we ask for. So does James. In chapter 4 verse 2-8 he wrote this:

> "<u>You lust and do not have</u>. You murder and covet and cannot obtain. You fight and war. Yet you do not have because you do not ask. ³You **ask and do not receive, because you ask amiss**, that you may <u>spend it on your pleasures</u>. ⁴Adulterers and adulteresses! Do you not know that friendship with the world is (to be an enemy) with God? Whoever therefore wants to be a friend of the world makes himself an enemy of God. ⁵Or do you think that the Scripture says in vain, "The Spirit who dwells in us yearns jealously?" ⁶But He gives more grace. Therefore He says:
>
> "God resists the proud,
>
> but gives grace to the humble."
>
> ⁷Therefore submit to God. Resist the devil and he will flee from you. ⁸Draw near to God and He will draw near to you. Cleanse your hands, you sinners; and purify your hearts, you doubleminded."

If our asking is for the wrong reasons (if our motives aren't pure) or if we do not ask according to God's will, then we will not receive what we ask for. And, yes, you can and should know God's will. Verse 8 speaks to how we do that, but admittedly that requires some effort on our part.

Do you want to live free from habits? Do you want to achieve stellar victories in life? Do you want to walk in health and see great power operating in your life? Do you want to have freedom in your food choices and still live a long and prosperous life? Then you <u>must</u> change the way you see the world and your relationship to it.

Hebrews 11:6 says very plainly:

> "But <u>without faith</u> it is **impossible** to please Him,
> for he who comes to God must believe that He is,
> and that He is a rewarder of those who <u>diligently</u>
> <u>seek Him</u>." (Emphasis added.)

In order to please God we must walk in faith. Now this faith is not that generic faith that we often hear some new celebrity talk about. "Oh, you've just got to have faith," they gush as they discuss their sudden rise from obscurity to the spotlight. They may even give a nod to God, but what they really mean is you have to have faith in yourself, and fate, and the world, and the fact that if you're just a good person things will work out.

This is also not the faith of just anyone believing in just any religion. This faith being discussed here has a definite root and source. First, the root of this faith is God himself, as the scriptures tell us:

> "For I say, through the grace given to me, to
> **everyone** who is among you, not to think of

himself more highly than he ought to think, but to think soberly, as God has dealt (given) to each one a measure of faith." (Romans 12:3)

Second, the source is the word of God:

"So then faith comes by hearing, and hearing by the word of God." (Romans 10:17)

What we can see, if we allow ourselves to see, is that the faith that pleases God is that faith which is provided by God and nurtured through His word. (Romans 12:3) Now, when we say it is provided by God, what that means is that every person who receives Christ does so by hearing the word and faith is intiated or deposited in their heart to believe on Him. We know this is so as we look at the passage in Romans 10. If we look to verses 8, 9 and 10 we see that the discussion centers in how a person is saved.

"⁸But what does it say? "The word is near you, in your mouth and in your heart" (that is, the word of faith which we preach): ⁹that if you confess with your mouth the Lord Jesus and believe in your heart that God has raised Him from the dead, you will be saved. ¹⁰For with the heart one believes unto righteousness, and with the mouth confession is made unto salvation."

We can see a further discussion of this in the following verses:

¹³For "whoever calls on the name of the LORD shall be saved." ¹⁴How then shall they call on Him in whom they have not believed? And how shall

they believe in Him of whom they have not
heard? And how shall they hear without a
preacher? (Romans 10:13-14)

The message of these verses is; the hearing of the word is that
which initiates faith in the heart of a person to believe on Jesus
as Lord and Savior. If the word is not preached then no one hears
and there is little to initiate faith. [Fortunately for mankind God
has also seen fit to reveal to the heart of every man, the fact that
He exists and that there is a coming judgment and that we all
need Him to escape it, (see Romans 1:18-20). This knowledge
does not normally initiate faith but can initiate a seeking by the
person who responds to it. A preacher, or a witness, is usually
still required to bring that person to the true and living God.]

In Romans 1:15-17 Paul discusses what portion of the word
we are to preach to the world that they may hear, have faith initiated and take action on. He said;

"15So, as much as is in me, *I am* ready to preach
the gospel to you who are in Rome also.16For I
am not ashamed of the gospel of Christ, for it is
the power of God to salvation for everyone who
believes, for the Jew first and also for the Greek.
17For in it the righteousness of God is revealed
from faith to faith; as it is written, "The just shall
live by faith." "

*   *   *

Fully pleasing God does not equal being fully loved by God.

Before we continue on this theme of living by faith let me provide a caveat, or a qualification. The idea of pleasing God does <u>not</u> mean that we have to perform a certain way or do certain things in order for God to love us. The God who **is** love (1 John 4:8, 16) simply loves us because that is His nature. He loved us so much that He sent His Son to die to restore mankind's relationship with Him (John 3:16). Jesus went about "doing good and healing all who were oppressed of the devil" (Acts 10:38) in order to demonstrate God's love for us. It is not our performance that pleases God in the traditional sense of the word "pleases." God is pleased with us right now and for all time because He is pleased with Jesus and the saved, or born again, believer is **in Christ**. We are seated with Him in heavenly places (Ephesians 2:4-6), we have been made new creatures in Christ (2 Corinthians 5:17; Galatians 6:14), and the list goes on.

Jesus became the "propitiation" for our sins (Romans 3.25; Hebrews 2:17; 1 John 2:2; 4:10), which primarily means "satisfaction." God is satisfied by Jesus' sacrifice and the punishment He bore for our sins. However, we can "make God proud" so to speak when we obey Him. In fact, in one place He expressed specifically that obedience is better than (any) sacrifice (1 Samuel 15:22). As a parent I understand this, and for those of you who are parents if you will think on this you will get it, too.

Let me express it this way. When I tell my girls to do their chores while I am gone, I fully expect them to do so. I anticipate that when I come home I will find the house reasonably clean, the dishes done, the animals fed and the clothes folded. If, upon my arrival home, I find this is not the case then I am displeased. Now, my lack of pleasure may communicate itself in ways that God's lack of pleasure won't. I may get angry and bark at my kids a bit (a trait I am overcoming), however there is no question I still love my children. There is also no question that the primary reason I am displeased is because everyone in the house suffers when one of them fails to accomplish their tasks. It may not directly affect my other girls in that they may not have to listen to my lecture or have to redo any chores, but they are affected because my attention is diverted and given to resolving the situation.

Later, the one who didn't perform may come to me and offer me a hug or some other expression of love. While I appreciate these expressions, a much greater expression in this situation would have been to complete the tasks given to them. However, while they may lose some privileges as a result of not doing their tasks they do not lose their "rights". I still provide a home, clothing, food, attention, activities, comforts, love, affection and a caring heart.

As I alluded to previously, I am not a perfect example because my own flesh can get into the mix but God is perfect. His reaction to our failure to perform will not be condemnation, but there may be a rebuke.

What happens when God directs your attention to a scripture that provides a rebuke for some action in your life? First, of course, is that sense that we "let Him down," but immediately thereafter we should come to that place that we realize what He expects of us and our hearts should be encouraged (see Hebrews 12:12-13). The Word of God should once again begin to produce faith. Of course the chastening, or rebuke, isn't pleasant but God does not chasten you to humiliate you, He chastens you to move you on to a higher level of faith. Go with God on this, not with your emotional response to your thoughts of failure. Pick yourself up, dust yourself off and begin to follow God once more.

We live in a time of sound bites, microwaves and speed-to-shelf, and it is increasingly difficult to understand that God does not relate to us in this hasty fashion. I don't mean that He doesn't have times when He directs you to do something within a deadline that may crunch you a bit. What I mean is that in order for us to really know God what is required is time studying to know God. We live in a hurry up society, but God says, *"Be still and know that I am God."* (Psalm 46:10) He desires that you turn off the tube, pull your earphones out of your ears and sit down in a quiet place. Not for a few so-called "quality" minutes, but for a quantity of quality minutes.

Relating to God is very much like relating to your best friend, or your spouse. You have to spend some time together finding out what He says, how He thinks, and how He acts. The difference is, you can't do that exactly the same way because God isn't human, He is a Spirit, and they that worship Him **must** worship Him in spirit and truth (John 4:24).

To reiterate, the "problem" we are having in life today is our way of thinking. We spend too much time listening to CNN, CBN, Newsweek, USA Today, doctors, nutritionists and dietitians and not enough time truly *listening to* God, through His Word. If we begin to listen more to God, we will grow in our understanding and our faith. This will enable us to respond to God's, rather than men's, opinion of our condition. In other words, we'll begin to think like Him.

Chapter Four

What the New Testament Says about Food

The New Testament has poignant and telling things to say regarding our food choices. Not things about specific foods, but things about how we are to receive our food and who we are to permit judging us with regard to our food. There are also admonitions regarding our attitude about our food choices.

Romans 13 beginning at verse 10 tells us that the important issue in our lives is to walk in the light, beginning with *"Love does no harm to a neighbor therefore love is the fulfillment of the law."* From there we are instructed to wake up, cast off the works of darkness and put on the "armor of light" which is not physical armor, but the very nature and personality of Christ. He is our salvation, our righteousness, the truth, our faith ("we live by the faith of the Son of God," Galatians 2:22) and He is the Word—both *logos* (the complete expression) and *rhema* (the specific word for a moment)—of God. Putting on the armor, as expounded by Paul in Ephesians 6, is synonymous with *"but put on the Lord Jesus Christ, and make no provision for the flesh, to fulfill its lusts."* (Romans 13:14)

This book is not written to create strife, or to gain any provision for my own flesh, such as an excuse to eat whatever I want or to behave in any manner I please. My desire and intent is to relieve those who have been burdened by unnecessary "laws" and requirements for Christian living that keep us from realizing the full potential of "Christ in us, the hope of Glory."

Although Romans 13 says love doesn't harm a neighbor and chapter 14 of Romans explains the importance of not doing things that offend just for the sake of your own self-satisfaction, the instruction not to offend pertains **not** to "political correctness" whereby we all must figure out what words *might* offend someone and then refrain from saying those things. In fact, we are not even to go around avoiding offending certain groups. Jesus said He did not come to bring peace, but a sword (albeit not the sword of terror). Some people are offended as a natural response to our faith. The gospel and the attendant life-instructions are offensive to all those who choose not to believe, because it challenges their own belief system. In fact, it calls them to face the fact that there is a God (Romans 1:18-21), and they are without God and without hope in this world,

(Ephesians 2:12). They have suppressed the truth in unrighteousness (Romans 1:18) and thus when the truth is presented, their desire is to silence that truth lest they become convicted and have to change.

For a believer taking a stand against sin does not usually mean taking a stand against the people engaged in that sin. Jesus often demonstrated His love for people **without condoning** their sin. In fact, in the case of the woman taken in the act of adultery (John 8:1-11), Jesus demonstrated mercy without breaking the law by declaring that the one who was without sin among them should cast the first stone. He also demonstrated grace when none there could pass that test save He. He told the woman neither did He condemn her, but he also added, **"Go and sin no more."**

To the man who was healed at the pool of Bethesda he instructed, "Sin no more, lest a worse thing come upon you." And that reveals God's primary issue with sinful acts that we commit, that our sins destroy us! It is not that God can't endure sin. In fact, Jesus came and lived among sinners. It is that God, Jesus and the Holy Spirit understand how very destructive sin is to us. We kid ourselves when we think that there are "victimless" crimes such as prostitution. The woman or man engaging in sexual acts outside the realm of marriage as described in Genesis is inviting all kinds of hellish activity into their lives.

Considering the fact that Paul instructed us to walk properly (Romans 13:13) *"as in the day, not in orgies and drunkenness, not in lewdness and lust, not in strife and jealousy.* [14]*But put on the Lord Jesus Christ...*" we should realize that the issues in chapter Fourteen concerning food are not major issues.

Where food becomes a major issue is when people begin to attempt to pervert the word for their own purposes, or when the world begins to express that the hope of long-life lies in eating one thing and not eating another.

Life is not lived long by those who simply control their diet, or who exercise, or those who do or don't drink alcohol. Even those who eat right, exercise and take what Paul told Timothy to do as a recommendation for them (1 Timothy 5:22) can be struck down by a bus, a plane crash, a hurricane, a tornado, a terrorist, a car accident or one of their fellow men or women. Life is not guaranteed to those who "do the right things." Life is guaranteed to those who live for Christ.

I can say that life is guaranteed to those who live for Christ because in Him we have eternal life. Eternal life is first of all, knowing God and knowing His Son Jesus Christ (John 17:3). Second, it is a life of abundance in Christ (John 10:10). Third, eternal life is living forever with the Lord (John 3:16).

For me, abundant living means not spending most of my time determining what I can or can't eat, or fixing carefully only those specific foods I am allowed. I am a husband and father of four, with a full life. My wife does homeschool for three of our four girls while taking care of the home as well as exercising and participating in our church. She has friends and family whom she ministers to and/or enjoys their company. We do not desire to be encumbered by dietary requirements that are expensive in either time or money. Thus we choose foods at times, for their convenience as opposed to the nutritional value they are deemed to hold by earthly people.

Paul said this, *"For one believes he may eat all things, but he who is weak eats only vegetables."* (Romans 14:2) Later in the chapter he stated, "I know and am convinced by the Lord Jesus that *there is* nothing unclean of itself; but to him who considers anything to be unclean, to him *it is* unclean."

In Colossians chapter two Paul wrote, *"So let no one judge you in food or in drink, or regarding a festival or a new moon or sabbaths, which are a shadow of things to come, but the substance is of Christ"* (vv. 16-17), and in 1 Corinthians he said if we partake of our food with thanksgiving then why are we criticized or judged for that which we eat? (1 Corinthians 10:30)

There is no doubt that we have many different camps in the world regarding diet and exercise, but it is time for all of us to realize that we are not master over another. The only master of a believer should be Jesus, and each of us should stand only before Him with regard to issues that are not specifically sin. Of course, Romans 13 instructs us to obey those governing bodies of men as long as they do not oppose God or godly principles. This extends to our jobs and schools and etc. The comment regarding only one master pertains to our individual choices. However, even our individual choices must come under the heading of Romans 13:10 *"Love does no harm to a neighbor; therefore love is the fulfillment of the law,"* and as Paul expounded specifically with regard to food in chapter 14 of Romans. Our heart must lead us to avoid intentional offense in specific instances. If I dine with a vegan brother who firmly believes that any who eat meat cannot be saved, and if my eating meat in front of my brother causes him to lose confidence in *his* salvation or prevents us from being able to fellowship, I should not eat that meat. However, if not eating meat is simply surrender to someone else's control of my life and does not threaten that individual's trust in God then I should come under the bondage of no one.

That returns us to what Paul said in 1 Corinthians; why do I have to be subject to being criticized simply to satisfy someone else's desire to be right or to have control. While I may avoid specific foods, or words, or actions in front of such a person to maintain peace in that moment; I will not allow myself to have to live under that person's control or judgment. I will live under the direction of the Lord through the Holy Spirit. If the Lord directs me not to eat certain foods or read certain books, etc. then I should obey His specific direction for me.

If you want to eat ice cream, steak, or Taco Bell, and you have no specific restrictions from the Lord for you, receive it with thanks and trust God that He causes what you eat to be sanctified (or separated) to your body and that it will sustain you. Don't take vitamins because people show you studies that declare how much of a deficit your body must have. Don't eat vegan because someone declares that killing animals is inhumane, don't avoid fast food because everyone tells you it isn't good for you.

If you are going to take vitamins or eat only vegetables, or cut out red meat from your diet, you must do so "from faith." Romans 14:23 tells us, "…whatever is not from faith is sin." Faith is confidence in what God has said. Some have found certain places in the Bible where it seems to teach that we must eat a certain way and their faith is placed in that, and they should follow those restrictions or guidelines. But faith is not faith if it is confidence in what someone *said God said*. In fact, that is one of the issues involved in Eve's temptation. She did not know for herself what God had said, for if she had she would not have misquoted Him, and she would not have been seduced into rejecting Him.

In 1 Timothy chapter 4 Paul is giving instructions regarding the "latter times" (v. 1). In the latter times, which we are living in, people will be *"speaking lies in hypocrisy … forbidding to marry, **and** commanding to abstain from foods … received with thanksgiving by those who believe and know the truth. For every creature … is good, and nothing is to be refused if … received with thanksgiving, for it is sanctified …."* (VV. 2-5) In verse 6 he says if you teach people about these "lies in hypocrisy" then you are a good minister. If you tell people that marriage is godly and eating foods received with thanksgiving is good because it is sanctified by the word of God and prayer, then you are doing what is good before God.

New Testament guidelines clearly permit far more foods than many people would have us believe. Remember, though, permission always relates to your faith. If you do not think or believe

37

you may eat certain foods, or do without certain supplements, than you should not. However, it is time for you to invest in knowing God's word accurately and completely, that you may change your thinking regarding foods and even all of life. Don't limit God's work in your life by limiting your thought process to the way you've always been.

Chapter Five

Synergy: Old Testament Principles in a New Testament World

Where do I begin, to tell the story...?

The Old Testament is filled with verses that speak directly to food and many that indirectly relate to the dietary laws. The first verse presented by many who want to direct your eating habits and food choices is the verse in Genesis 1:29: *"God said, "See, I have given you every herb that yields seed which is on the face of all the earth, and every tree whose fruit yields seed; to you it shall be for food."*

Related verses in Daniel chapter 1 and particularly verse 12 that says, *"Please test your servants for ten days, and let them give us vegetables to eat and water to drink."*

These verses, and more, have often been presented as the argument for eating primarily or exclusively vegetables. Let me remind you, though, that Paul stated that, "he who is weak eats (only) vegetables." While eating vegetables has been recognized as a beneficial food choice for generations, it is not the only food choice. I enjoy fruits and vegetables but not all fruits or vegetables. I am grateful that I may choose to eat some and not others while not risking my health any more than any person walking the planet today.

There are a limited number of people who would advocate a so-called biblical approach to vegetarianism because even casual Bible students are aware that God altered the diet plan by providing meats after Noah and his family left the Ark. Genesis 9:3 says, *"Every moving thing that lives shall be food for you. I have given you all things, even as the green herbs."* If you read the 9th chapter there is no way to confuse the above quotation. God was including every single animal, reptile and even insect as a potential food choice for them.

For the next several hundred years there were **no restrictions** on what food they ate, except that they did not eat meat with the blood. God did not distinguish between clean animals and unclean regarding food until the coming of the law. There was a distinction when they loaded the ark and when they sacrificed to the Lord, but not in regard to their diet.

It was only at the giving of the law that God gave specifics and defined clean and unclean animals with regard to food choices (Leviticus 20:25). Only with the giving of the law did he tell them not to eat fat (Leviticus 3:17; 7:23). However, in

Nehemiah 8:10, following the reading of the law to these Jews who had been away from it for so many years, they were told to "Eat the fat, drink the sweet," and save portions for those who were not present or who had none. I can only conclude that the prohibition against eating the fat pertained specifically to sacrificial animals. Many of the sacrifices that were made were shared with the Priests and Levites while the remainder was consumed by the family. The fat was always to be burned in the sacrifice. Once again evidence that attempting to take specific scriptures from the Old Testament and use them as specific rules for the way we are required to eat is actually inappropriate.

One book I read was written by a doctor who is a spirit-filled believer. He is well known and definitely has some insightful things to say with regard to healing. In the book he draws attention to such points as; it was God's original health plan that we not get sick. He also says, on page 92 of his book, "Dwelling in you is the healing, life-giving Spirit of God. The Word goes forth, healing and delivering us from <u>our</u> destructions. There are some hindrances—like sin, bondage, rebellion and doubt—that block this divine flow from coming out of our spirit man and into our bodies." (The Doctor and the Word; 1996; Creation House.)

I believe that the sentence regarding any hindrance defines the heart of the matter and is just one of several insightful points the doctor makes. However, in his writing he also includes things that are not completely accurate regarding the nature and character of God. The mission of this book is not to critique any specific book. Neither is it to criticize any individual in a harmful way. As I have stated, the purpose in writing this is to present the grace of God as related to our food choices. There will be specific challenges made to some statements made by others, but only for the purpose of bringing light onto this subject.

I must begin again with further comments made by the author of the above mentioned book. In this book the author states that God's original plan (which I agree with) was not supernatural healing but that we never get sick. He reasons that God presented the "covenant of healing" to a people who were not even sick (Exodus 15:26) and then goes on to state that God gave them dietary laws immediately after this. Upon reading the chapter of Exodus, and those following, you will see that it was not "immediately" that God gave dietary laws. What's more, when God gave them dietary laws he also gave them laws with regard to nearly every facet of life. Laws that were designed to reflect the separation between natural and spiritual, and laws that were designed to demonstrate that man cannot achieve relationship with God by *doing*.

That being the case it becomes problematic to assume that Jesus fulfilled some laws and not all. It was stated that the "ceremonial laws" that were types of Jesus were fulfilled but that the moral laws, such as the Ten Commandments, still apply today. If that be true then the punishments associated with those laws must also continue. Quickly, before you burn me in effigy let me qualify that.

We are not under the law of adultery or murder or stealing or coveting, which are found in the Ten Commandments as it pertains to God. These laws were given in the Old Testament because man had come to a place in which he was interpreting a lack of judicial activity on God's part as a license to define right and wrong (see Genesis 4:23-24 and Lamech's speech.)

As Genesis moves forward from Lamech God expresses His displeasure with the attitude of man, and it must be concluded that much of that attitude was expressed by Lamech in his speech. Here are his words, "I am more righteous than Cain because I killed in self-defense, so surely God will justify me even more than Cain." You can find this same attitude expressed today in statements such as, "what goes around, comes around. If you do good, then you'll be rewarded." People often compare what they do with what their friends and neighbors do and determine that they're okay, which is precisely what Lamech was doing.

Paul warned against this in 2 Corinthians 10:12.

"For we dare not class ourselves or compare
ourselves with those who commend themselves.
But they, measuring themselves by themselves,
and comparing themselves among themselves,
are not wise."

Prior to the flood debauchery reigned unchecked, and mankind was determined to justify themselves by their own standards. By the time God expresses His displeasure with man's

43

attitude, as we all know, Noah was one of very few righteous remaining on the earth. By the time of the flood, Noah may have been the only righteous person. (Methuselah was alive and well when God called Noah to build the ark. He didn't die until the year of the flood. He was a righteous man.) Now, this begs the question, what was it that Noah did that made him righteous?

The Word provides the answer in Genesis 6:9 "Noah was a just man, perfect in his generations. Noah **walked with** God." (Emphasis added) There is further evidence of this found in Hebrews 11:7.

> "By faith Noah, being divinely warned of things not yet seen, moved with godly fear, prepared an ark for the saving of his household, by which he condemned the world and became heir of the righteousness which is according to faith."

In other words, it is not what Noah did, but what Noah believed that made the difference. Certainly it is recorded that he *did* things, but those things were an expression of what he believed, of his response to what God said to him. In contrast, it was also not what all the others *did* that condemned them. Rather it was, "*that* every intent of the thoughts of (their) heart *was* only evil continually." (Genesis 6:5b)

The laws were given not to provide man a means of righteousness or a method by which he could or should maintain health. They were given to demonstrate that man, in his own ability, did not have the capability to live up to God's perfect standard. God was not using that standard up to the time of the law, which included several hundred years after Noah and the Ark, in which God continued to deal with Mankind through mercy and grace. (*"For <u>until the law</u> sin was in the world, but sin is <u>not imputed</u> **when there is no law.** [14]Nevertheless death reigned from Adam to Moses, even over those who had not sinned according to the likeness of the transgression of Adam, who is a type of Him who was to come,"* Romans 5:13-14.) However, once again, man began to demonstrate the same propensity toward self-destructive, fleshly activities as were present at the time of the flood. Thus, God gave the law to restrain the effects of sin and show man his inability to save himself.

As a side point, the law was given to restrain the effects of sin. In other words, you can legislate morality to a large degree. If you could not then why would we have laws pertaining to murder and stealing and drunk driving? Many opponents of order and the rule of law argue that by making things illegal we only encourage people to "sample the forbidden fruit." On the contrary, while some are encouraged in that way, the existence of the law deters most from "sampling." But I digress.

In the giving of the law God made a distinction between those who would follow after Him and those who would be heathen or gentiles. The purpose was to reveal man's inability to be righteous *and* to preserve the righteous line, in order to bring Jesus into the earth to accomplish His plan.

The Old Testament provides examples for us and relates principles that form the basis of our walk with God, but the Old Testament, while a true revelation of God, is also an incomplete revelation. Without the window of the New Testament we cannot see into the complete nature and character of God. Once we do begin our exploration via the New Testament than we can enjoy our study of the Old Testament and our opportunity to learn from the examples, good and bad, that are recorded.

Chapter Six

Reconciling

It has been said there are three kinds of people in the world. First there are stupid people who don't learn from their mistakes, repeating them again and again. Second there are smart people who do learn from their own mistakes. Third there are wise people, they learn from other people's mistakes. Don't just be smart, be wise!

I stated at the close of the last chapter that the Old Testament provides examples. This is recorded in the New Testament and is not something I theorized on my own. *"Now all these things happened to them as examples, and they were written for our admonition, upon whom the ends of the ages have come."* (1 Corinthians 10:11)

We can study the lives of Old Testament characters, be they

believer or non-believer, and learn to avoid many of life's pit-falls. For instance, Joseph is a wonderful example of how a believer should act when facing adversity. Armed only with a dream from God and no written scripture, Joseph lived a life of integrity, honor, service and character that is not often emulated. In slavery, in prison, in the dungeon slaving for other prisoners, made no difference to Joseph. He did not complain, he did not give up and he did not give in to temptation. He continually did the "right thing" before God. Would that I could say that I have always had such a testimony.

Though I can't say I have always managed adversity the way Joseph did, I thoroughly believe that a thoughtful study of his life and a steady diet of thinking about the lessons found in it would have enabled me to produce that type of character earlier in my life.

The example was there for me, if only I had taken the time to do as Joshua 1:8 instructs me, or Psalm 1:2; if I had taken the time to "meditate" on these lessons night and day I would have avoided some of those embarrassing moments that come when you are just whining and feeling sorry for yourself, and everyone knows it. Not to mention how much more I would have limited the enemy's activity in my life and instead, released God's power.

I can't do anything about what is past, as you can't, but we can determine to follow the instructions of the two references above and learn from the lives of those who have gone before.

Of course, this chapter is about reconciling Old and New thus

I am compelled to point out that Romans 12:1-3 gives instruction similar to Joshua and Psalms.

> "I beseech you therefore, brethren, by the mercies of God, that you present your bodies a living sacrifice, holy, acceptable to God, which is your reasonable service. ²And **do not be conformed** to this world, but <u>be transformed</u> by the <u>renewing of your mind</u>, that you may prove what is that good and acceptable and perfect will of God.
> ³For I say, through the grace given to me, to everyone who is among you, <u>not to think</u> of *himself* more highly than he ought to think, but to <u>think soberly</u>, as God has dealt to each one a measure of faith." (Emphasis added.)

We are to "be transformed" in thought, character, and conduct, by "renewing...(the) mind." That renewing does not come by thinking the same old thoughts. I stated at the beginning of the book that self-help gurus and psychologists agree that we must alter our thinking in order to alter our behaviors. However, we must alter our thinking based on what God has said.

We reconcile Old Testament instructions and principles with New Testament doctrine by first being well-versed in what the New Testament has to say. I have supplied numerous verses that pertain to the topic at hand and a thorough study of these and surrounding verses provide the foundation by which you can then read and understand the lessons provided in the Old Testament, and provide the tools for meditation and altering your thinking.

Daniel's call for only vegetables and water can be seen as a means of living a fasted lifestyle, rather than a specific set of instructions regarding food choices, when we understand that Paul denounces eating "only vegetables" as being weak in faith. We can also recognize that restrictions on clean and unclean animals had specific application to the time in which the law was given, but has been fulfilled the same as all of the law since Jesus came.

A fasted lifestyle as expressed by Daniel's request, and as demonstrated by Paul's life, is a lifestyle that simply does not allow the flesh to have everything it thinks it wants. Paul said it this way in 1 Corinthians 9:27, *"But I discipline my body and bring it into subjection, lest, when I have preached to others, I myself should become disqualified."*

Limiting our food intake, or limiting our television viewing, or even limiting our working hours, are forms of fasting, provided you use them to "discipline (your) body and bring it into subjection." By that I mean that you use those times to focus more on God's word, either directly through reading and studying it, or indirectly by thinking and meditating on it. As you deny your flesh, and nourish your soul in Godly things, you will be "transformed" in your thinking which will result in different actions.

Remember, Einstein's definition of insanity is, "doing the same thing and expecting a different result." I have a coin inscribed this way, "If you always do what you've always done, you will always be what you've always been."

Proverbs 23:7 says, *"As a man* (or woman) *thinks in* (the) *heart so is he*/**she**." You are the product of what you think on, and your actions do reflect those thoughts. You can change, but you have to change the thoughts first, and those changes must be guided by what God has said or it is just more sowing to the flesh. (Galatians 6:8 *For he who sows to his flesh will of the flesh reap corruption, but he who sows to the Spirit will of the Spirit reap everlasting life.*)

The Bible, Genesis to Revelation, is a complete revelation of the will of God, of the nature and character of God. In all the Bible there are truths that are enough to provide a person access into God's way of thinking and give them success in life. Joshua 1:8 says, *"This Book of the Law shall not depart from your mouth, but you shall meditate in it day and night, that you may observe to do according to all that is written in it. For then you will make your way prosperous, and then you will have good success."* God told him to meditate in the "Book of the Law." This was the first five books of the Bible we have today. God said there was enough truth in those books to give Joshua success.

Quickly, now, before anyone says I am countering my own arguments, let me add this does not mean all of the Truth is contained in those first five books. A person who knows how to add, subtract, multiply and divide has enough math skills to accomplish a significant number of tasks and enough to become prosperous and successful. They do not, however, have enough knowledge to build a submarine or a spaceship and explore realms where few other men go. For those things a more complete revelation of mathematics is required. The building blocks of advanced calculus lie in add, subtract, multiply and divide. These are the foundation. They are not calculus, thermodynamics or geometry, which are all required to build that ship

In the same way, the foundation of all we believe is found in Genesis and there is sufficient revelation waiting to provide success, however the secrets of that revelation are more readily unlocked as I use the tools of the New Testament. Jesus and Paul declared that the age in which we live is comprised of a mystery that was hidden in ages past. (Mark 4:11-12; Romans 16:25; 1 Corinthians 2:7-8; Ephesians 3:3-9) The Greek word they used to describe this mystery was; μυστεριον (musterion). This word describes something that is hidden to the uninitiated. He also stated that spiritual things can only be understood by means of the Spirit of God (Romans 8:7; Romans 16:25; 1 Corinthians 1:18). In other words they are **revealed**, not discovered or created.

Old Testament scripture contained all the elements of this Mystery, but were not intuitively obvious to a casual observer. Men like Samuel, David, Daniel and the prophets received glimpses into these truths but without the "key" it was very difficult to understand the "code." The key is passing through Jesus by means of the New Birth and being joined to the family of God (John 3:3-8; John 1:12-13) with the Holy Spirit being the connector. Then as you read the word and (and this is an extremely important "and") meditate in it, He, the Holy Spirit, will begin to teach you (John 14:26; 15:26; 16:13). In doing so He will compare scripture with scripture, rather than letting you have "creative ideas."

These two paragraphs have a huge amount of material packed into them and would require another book to properly explore. Take time to look at the references and listen to the Teacher. Meanwhile, as God leads and preferably in this order, study the epistles, study the gospels, study the lives of the Old Testament characters and study the Prophets. In all of this studying don't leave out Psalms and Proverbs for they are packed with insight. Look at the Bible, Genesis to Revelation, as a large tapestry. It has a picture of God and all the parts fit together. Sometimes you walk up close and really scrutinize part of it, and other times you back away to see how that part you were studying will fit into the whole. And it does fit if you look at it in context and with the help of the Holy Spirit.

In pursuing your studies there are many capable, anointed teachers to whom you can listen. I recommend three: Pastor Bob Yandian of Grace Fellowship Church in Tulsa, Oklahoma. You can find him on the web at www.precepts.com. And Andrew Wommack, of Colorado Springs, CO. You can find him at www.awmi.net.

Joyce Meyer is another good resource and she is at www.joycemeyer.org.

Chapter Seven

God Speaks to You!
Personal Convictions
and Specific Instructions

In spite of the fact that the Bible provides us guidance and direction for nearly all things there are some things that are not specifically covered. While there are scriptures that tell us how we are to conduct ourselves in the affairs of life, there are no scriptures that tell us specifically what career field to enter or where we are to live or who to marry, etc. Additionally, there are things that may be acceptable for one person but are specifically forbidden for another.

I had a friend who told me about a man he went to Bible school with. He said this man had been a great basketball player and really loved basketball. He would rather be playing hoops than anything else. It was like a god to him. When he got born again and committed his life to the Lord he gave up basketball entirely. It was not a specific direction from the Lord but a personal conviction on his part. He felt that it distracted him from his relationship with the Lord because of the amount of time and energy he was prone to give to basketball so he put it aside in favor of a deeper relationship with the Lord.

When I learned of this conviction I was not moved in any way to give up basketball. I've played basketball for most of my life and enjoyed the game. I did not spend excessive hours on the court and I do not watch it on TV very often. For me, basketball has been a part of my life and an opportunity to hang with other guys, not an idol. I have recently stopped playing basketball because it interfered with running and a balanced life. I have gotten into running long distances both for fitness and as a means of ministry. Running and basketball can be compatible but in my case they are not. I have a wife and four children and other responsibilities. Trying to run and play basketball would require far too much time and would be irresponsible, <u>for me</u>.

These are just two examples of personal convictions that are derived from a foundation of the scripture. For the basketball player verses such as Matthew 6:33 and Joshua 1:8 came into play. He felt he would not be spending enough time meditating in the word, or in seeking **first** the Kingdom if he continued to play basketball because it was an obsession with him.

In my case, I believe that ministering to runners is part of my calling but so is loving and serving my family. I feel I would not do either adequately if I throw in another sport.

In some cases, a personal conviction may change as you grow. The basketball player may one day find that he can hang with some guys and "shoot hoops" again without it becoming an obsession. I may find that as our church grows an overall sports program fits in with our core efforts. If so, I may find myself playing basketball sometimes, or softball, or soccer, or who knows.

By the same token, there are things in all of our lives that are not good for us, that have a bit of control over our flesh. We may recognize through our time with the Lord, or through the times we tend to avoid time with the Lord, that these things are not profitable for us. We may then choose to put those down in our lives. Those are personal convictions and if they are not specifically prohibited as sin in the Bible they are not doctrines to be preached to others. It may be that you relate your choice to someone and they agree with it and follow suit but that does not mean that everyone must.

In the same vein, there are things that God may specifically direct a person NOT to do or eat or wear, or a place they should not go. In James we're told that the man who knows to do right and does not do it, to him it is sin. (James 4:16) When God specifically directs someone not to eat meat, or to not eat certain foods they should not. However, they are not at liberty to preach that as a doctrine from God. They may share the "why and where for" of their decision and others may recognize a witness in their own hearts that leads them to the same conclusion, but that still does not make it doctrine for all.

We used to watch a certain television show every Wednesday night. In 2003 I was spending time seeking the Lord and He directed me to not watch that show that season. Watching TV together was something my wife and I have done since we married in 1986. Sometimes we each watched shows just to be with each other although one or the other of us didn't prefer a particular show. It was a bit challenging to me to stay away from the living room during that hour on Wednesdays since it is the hub of our house. But I had a specific direction from the Lord that I was to spend time with Him during that hour.

I would often spend more than that hour as a result but only that hour was specifically directed by God. My wife did not join me, nor did I suggest or demand that she do so. That specific direction was for me and it was for me to spend time with the Lord.

Subsequently I no longer sensed a specific direction regarding that time and that show. I have not watched it nearly as much as I once did for various reasons but I believe part of the reason was that during that season I lost my "taste" for the show. Less TV can only be a good thing, so now following my personal conviction and not watching the show does not harm me in any way. I would recommend that choice to everyone however it is my personal conviction. Spending less time in natural pursuits and more with the Lord is definitely general direction from the word of God but how you do that is between you and God.

Another personal conviction of mine convinces me that there is benefit in following some of the guidelines provided by people such as Dr. Cherry. I believe as an athlete there are some things I can do to enhance my performance both in training and in nutrition. However, I believe that much of that derives from my own affirmation of these things.

The Jews ate manna and quail for 40 years in the wilderness. Elijah out ran a chariot on the strength of some food cooked by an angel. David ate the showbread which, according to the law, was only for the priests, and he didn't die. Samson was sustained by honey alone at one time and Jesus fasted 40 days without croaking. In fact, Jesus informed the devil that "Man does not live by bread only, but by every word of God," when that dude tried to get Him to turn stones into bread. Something He was capable of doing, I believe, if his feeding more than 20,000 people with a few loaves and fish is any indication.

"Foods for the stomach and the stomach for foods, but God will destroy both it and them," 1 Corinthians 6:13 tells us. The body and its needs are not, and should not be, the primary driver in the lives of true followers of Jesus Christ because they will not last. Galatians 5:24 *"those who are Christ's have crucified the flesh with its passions and desires. 25If we live in the Spirit, let us also walk in the Spirit."*

Life is so much more than this earthly body and its base

desires. God understands this far better than we do. That is why there are times He gives a person specific directions or prohibitions. Following His direction or abiding by His prohibition is not limiting it is liberating. *"To obey is better than sacrifice,"* (1 Samuel 15:22). God would rather we obey than to make elaborate sacrifices, however our obedience frees us to enjoy all the blessings and benefits of the life He gives. If you look at the text in 1 Samuel 15 you will see that Saul did not completely obey God's instruction, to the point of rebellion, and as a result he lost his throne. It didn't happen immediately, but his anointing to be king was gone and from there it was a matter of time until the resultant loss of power and position, not to mention life. On the other hand obedience in that situation would have resulted in our hearing of the "sure mercies of Saul" and that Jesus would be the "son of Saul" instead of David.

It requires self-discipline to choose to obey God. The rewards are unfathomable and the consequences are also beyond our understanding until we live them. If you have specific direction from the Lord or your heart leads you to prohibit something in your life not necessarily prohibited by the Word, have the courage to obey. Enjoy the blessings of obedience but don't let others condemn you if you're not convicted about your diet. If you are one who is convicted regarding you're diet, don't attempt to bring condemnation on others who are not.

"Be it unto you according to your faith."

Chapter Eight

Discipline: What It Is; What It Is Not

I mentioned self-discipline as a requirement to obedience as we closed chapter seven. Self-discipline is not automatic. All self-discipline is introduced and developed by means of external discipline. Our parents, our teachers, our bosses and other leaders all imposed discipline on us. If we submitted to that external discipline we began to develop self-discipline. In the same way there is discipline in God's kingdom that can teach us to follow God willingly and with a ready heart.

The book of Hebrews tells us that God chastens, or disciplines, all His children and if He doesn't chasten you then you're not one of His kids (Hebrews 12:5-13). Jesus said that we should rebuke a brother (or sister) in the Lord, if they sin against us

(Luke 17:4). In 1 Timothy 5:20 Paul tells us to rebuke those who are sinning, and in 2 Timothy 4:2 he tells Timothy to, *"Preach the word! Be ready in season and out of season. Convince,* **rebuke,** *exhort, with all longsuffering and teaching."* Again, in Titus he instructs leaders to rebuke (Titus 1:13, 2:15). Finally, in Revelation 3:19 Jesus told John, *"As many as I love I rebuke and chasten."*

The "rod and rebuke" (Proverbs 29:15) that God uses is His word, that key document and guide book for life, not circumstances or sickness or tragedy. So often people believe that some great tragedy is God's method of whipping us instead of seeing those things for what they truly are. That cancer that is sucking the life out of you or your loved one is **not** a blessing from God sent to teach you anything.

Paul made it very clear in 2 Timothy that the Word, and the Word alone, is sufficient to bring us to maturity.

> "[16]<u>All Scripture</u> *is* given by inspiration of God, and *is* <u>profitable</u> for doctrine, for reproof, for correction, for instruction in righteousness, [17]that the man of God may be <u>complete, thoroughly equipped for every good work</u>." (2 Timothy 3:16-17).

It may be that you learn great things in adversity, but in life we usually call that the "school of hard knocks." This does not line up with the character of God as His instrument of instruction. Too many verses declare God's love, care and faithfulness. Yes, I know that many of those who preach this doctrine try to claim that it is because we just don't understand God's ways. "His ways are higher than our ways," they are fond of quoting. They are quoting from Isaiah 55:9; *"For as the heavens are higher than the earth, so are My ways higher than your ways, and My thoughts than your thoughts."* As you read this passage in context it is discussing how God desires to bless us as we seek Him. His passion is to "water" us with His word as the rain waters the ground, and for His word to perform the things He sends it for.

This passage in verse 9 regarding not knowing His ways, is a fact as long as your thoughts are of and from carnal things, i.e. the world, as Romans 8 says. However, even in the Old Testament God told the people to "come now and let us reason together," (Isaiah 1:18a). Even in this passage, He was saying we could gain insight into His ways. Psalms 119 is all about the Word and the benefits of knowing the Word. Take the time to read this Psalm and you will find numerous passages like, *"How can a young man cleanse his way? By taking heed according to your word."* (verse 9) or, *"Your word have I hidden in my heart that I might not sin against you."* (verse 11) Verse 17 says, *"Deal bountifully with your servant, that I may live and keep your word."* It is my contention that having a car accident, getting cancer, AIDS or some other terrible disease, or suffering from poverty are not things that make me think of the word "bountifully."

My contention finds its support in, once again, the New Testament. First, Acts 10:38 says, *"how God anointed Jesus of Nazareth with the Holy Spirit and with power, who went about doing good and* **healing all who were oppressed by the devil,** *for God was with Him.*" It is significant that, as we review the testimonies in the Gospels concerning Jesus, what we do not find is a single instance where He refused to heal someone because "it was God's will for them to be sick." Neither do we find Him ever saying some great tragedy was God's will.

There is one story in which a question was raised about a man born blind, and who had sinned to cause this. John 9:3, Jesus answered, *"Neither this man nor his parents sinned* (committed any specific act of sin), *but that the works of God should be revealed in him."* Many people point to this story and say, "see there, it was God's will." I beg to differ.

First, if God made this man blind Jesus would have been going against His will in healing the man. Second, God established in Deuteronomy 28 just where sickness and poverty come from. They are called "curses," not blessings from God. In fact, as you read through chapter 28 you find what the blessings are.

James supports this concept in the first chapter of his book, (1:13)

> "<u>Let no one say</u> when he is tempted, 'I am tempted by God'; for God cannot be tempted by evil, nor does He Himself tempt anyone. [14]But each one is tempted when he is drawn away by his own desires and enticed." (17) "Every good gift and every perfect gift is from above, and comes down from the Father of lights, with whom there is no variation or shadow of turning."

I don't know about you but cancer, car accidents, amputations and marital problems are not "good gifts" to me. Yes, I know that some who claim these are "God's will" suggest that since they are related to the physical body then we can't see them as being bad, we have to see them for what they produce in our lives. Well, if that were true then we have to come back to Jesus and ask why He never told anyone that. If a priest or minister is supposed to be His representative shouldn't they be saying what He said?

A thoughtful reading of Jesus' statement would show us that He is not explaining why the man was blind but stating that no matter the cause, God's glory would be revealed in his healing. Similarly, before He raised Lazarus from the dead He stated, *"This sickness is not unto death, but for the glory of God, that the Son of God may be glorified through it."* He was not stating what made Lazarus sick, rather He was explaining that God would receive glory when Lazarus was raised from the dead.

Jesus was also declaring in regard to the blind man, that some sicknesses occur not because of any specific sin, but because sin in general has entered the world and upset the perfect balance God created. (Romans 8:22; *For we know that the whole creation groans and labors with birth pangs together until now.*) Romans chapter 5 explains how the sin of Adam allowed death into the world, and all that attends death, meaning sickness, poverty, depression, pain, and even accidents. Sometimes, just because of the operation of sin in the world, bad things happen for no apparent reason. However, Jesus is declaring through these two cases that in all of that God is still greater and can turn cursing into blessing, or as Romans 8:28 says, He can work things together for our good.

That passage does **not** say all things are good for us, it says He can work all things, good and bad, together for our good.

Discipline. That is the topic of this chapter. What we've been dealing with is what God does not use to discipline us. I have already stated that what He does use is His Word. The Holy Spirit will use any voice He can to communicate the Word to you, to expose your disobedience that you may repent. In Numbers 22 God used a donkey to speak to Balaam. Balaam had become so hardened in his heart because of greed that he wasn't listening to God. Balaam already had God's answer concerning Balak and his cohorts. God told him **not** to go with them.

Balaam listened the first time, but when the men came back with more prominent celebrities Balaam was impressed. He was looking at outward things and thinking to himself, surely God didn't mean what He said. The Gold and the Glory beckoned him. He wanted to get paid, and he wanted to be recognized. He wanted to go to the hottest clubs and biggest parties and have everyone know his name. So when the second group came he went back to God and said, "Hey, did you really mean that?" God's answer was different but Balaam was missing something. God told him he could go but he'd better only say what God told him to say. Thing is, God answered Balaam the way Balaam hoped, but it was not what God first told Balaam to do. What's more, as Balaam went God had no confidence that he would say only what God told him to. He saw Balaam's hard-heartedness and God's anger came up. God sent the Angel of the Lord to ambush him.

Balaam's donkey had more spiritual perception than Balaam did. He saw this warrior Angel waiting and turned off the road. Balaam hit the donkey to get her back onto the road. A little farther down the Angel was waiting in a narrow alley and the donkey saw Him again. She scooted up close to one of the walls and smashed Balaam's foot. He hit her again. She headed up the road again but the Angel of the Lord had picked a new spot, waiting with His sword drawn in a narrow canyon in which there was no way to avoid Him. The donkey saw Him waiting and just plopped down on the road. Balaam hit her again, this time with his staff.

Finally God had his donkey speak. "Then the LORD opened the mouth of the donkey, and she said to Balaam, "What have I done to you, that you have struck me these three times?" (Numbers 22:28)

I don't know about you but if my car started talking to me I'd freak just a bit. Balaam didn't even miss a beat; he just began to argue with the donkey. 'And Balaam said to the donkey, "Because you have abused me. I wish there were a sword in my hand, for now I would kill you!"'

Balaam is furious and nearly out of his mind. This donkey talking to him doesn't get his attention. Amazingly the donkey's logic does. "So the donkey said to Balaam, '*Am* I not your donkey on which you have ridden, ever since *I became* yours, to this day? Was I ever disposed to do this to you?'" Balaam answered, "No." In that moment the significance of the situation penetrated his hard heart and he quit looking at the natural. As soon as he did his eyes were opened and he saw the Angel of the Lord standing before him, sword drawn ready to cut him down.

God was ready to slay Balaam for his sinful ways. Today, though, God has already slain someone for your sinful ways. Jesus was sacrificed to save you from sin and its consequences. His sacrifice was sufficient. God is **not** holding your sin against you. Don't misunderstand that. There are consequences of sin. Many are obvious. A promiscuous lifestyle may lead to AIDS or other STD's. Stealing or murder may bring incarceration or death. But results are not discipline.

If I drive too fast on the highway and get a ticket, that's a result. It may be discipline as far as the world sees it, but it is a result of my poor choice. God did not give me a ticket nor did He orchestrate it so I would get one. In fact, even the devil didn't give me a ticket. If I received a ticket it was because I was speeding and I was caught.

If I have a car accident that is a result. That may not be a result of a bad choice on my part. Perhaps I did everything right on the road but some other person ran a red light or a stop sign. God did not make that person run the stop sign and hit me and it may well be that the devil had nothing to do with it either. It is a result of living in a fallen world with sin and death trying to run rampant and many people cooperating with the same. That is not God's discipline. If that is how God disciplines then why would we consider it right to punish a parent who would inflict injury on a child in order to teach them?

If I want my child to avoid the hot stove I don't take her hand and place it on a hot burner, inflicting injury, and then tell her I did that because I love her and don't want her to get hurt. If I did that, I would rightly be branded a child abuser.

Discipline is defined in Webster's Deluxe Dictionary, Tenth Collegiate Edition as; *noun*; 4) training that corrects, molds, or perfects the mental faculties or moral character. 5) b: Orderly or prescribed conduct or pattern of behavior. 5) c: Self-control.

The first definition of Webster's for both the noun and verb have to do with punishment but we cannot apply that definition to God's discipline because first, Jesus was "punished" for us. Isaiah 53:4-6 tells us this, with verse 5b stating clearly, "The chastisement (whipping; punishment) for our peace *was* upon Him."

Second, the Greek word translated "chastisement" in Hebrews and other places is παιδευω (paideuo) and carries the definition; *to instruct, train, correct*; not to punish. This definition is in keeping with those I have quoted above and support the idea that God's discipline is designed to train and instruct us, to mold us into imitators of Him as a child imitates his father (*"Therefore be imitators of God as dear children."* Ephesians 5:1)

The book of Hebrews tells us that solid food belongs to those who by reason of use have their senses exercised to discern both good and evil. (Hebrews 5:14) "Senses exercised" means that a believer has spent time training their flesh that there is another sense other than the commonly recognized five senses. The other sense is faith. Faith is very simply a trust in something you can't see and even more a trust in what God has declared to be true even though it may contradict what your five senses tell you.

The truth is most of us are so dominated by our five senses that we would not know faith if it bit us in the backside. Not true Bible faith as described in Hebrews 11:1, *"Now faith is the substance of things hoped for, the evidence of things not seen."*

The "things not seen" part is what throws most people since that isn't compatible with "if I see it, then I'll believe it." That's what I mean about real Bible faith, a faith that has confidence that God's word is true even before I see any results. That's the kind of faith God wants me to have and that's the nature of the character He wants to mold in me. He does that through "discipline." He does that by instructing, training and correcting. He accomplishes those things by "the rod and rebuke."

In 1 Corinthians 13 Paul said we see "through a glass darkly" and James said that looking into the word is like looking into a mirror. The mirror reflects, but in this case, it reflects the nature and character of God. As we look into the word that Jesus said was "Spirit ... and life," we can see a reflection of His ways, of His will, and of His character. As we see these things our role is to begin to apply them to our lives so that we begin to change to look like that reflection. That is discipline. Pastor Nic Mihailoff defined discipline as "uncomfortable, yet long desired change produced by training, practice, coaching, parenting, etc."

Discipline is change. Discipline is change prompted by instruction or by training, but it is change that we embrace. As we embrace it we become self-disciplined through God's power. Not a self-control that brags but a self-control that responds to the Word and the Will of God.

I recently was sent a link on the internet called The Rope. Maybe some of you have seen this. It tells the tale of a man who was fit and strong and wanted to climb a mountain. In climbing he wanted it to be known that he had done this great thing himself; he wanted the glory. He asked for no help and began his ascent one morning. He climbed for hours, working his way up the mountain. The time passed and the hour grew late. He had not reached the peak before darkness set in but he was near. He switched on his head lamp and continued to climb.

He was reaching for a hand hold that was just at his limit. He pushed up on his foot hold, stretching for the grip when he suddenly slipped. He fell away from the wall and was hurling through the darkness, his head lamp beam waving around in the air. He could feel the slight tugs as each of his pitons, bolts and other aids popped free. His life rushed before his eyes. His heart raced. His body tensed, waiting for impact.

He felt the plunge slow, the yank on his harness was more substantial. Suddenly the headlong rush was stopped. His harness seized his mid-section as his rope finally held. The violent jerk caused his head lamp to fly off and he was swallowed in darkness. As he hung there he finally came to the end of himself.

"God, help me!"

In that moment he heard a voice. It was clear and distinct.

"What do you want me to do for you?"

"Please, save me!"

"Do you believe I can save you?"

"Yes, Lord. I believe you can do anything!"

"Then cut the rope that holds you."

The man was astonished. His mind instantly began to question the wisdom of such a thing. What was he supposed to think, that God would just catch him on a cloud, or with His hand? How could God ask him to cut the rope?

"Can't you see that the rope is my lifeline?" God spoke again, "The ground is near. Cut the rope." The man considered that. He stared down hard trying to see the ground. Too dark. He changed his body position several times trying to feel the ground. No good. Finally, the man decided that what God asked was foolish so he hung onto the rope.

The next day a search was mounted for the missing climber. He was finally found, unfortunately dead. The irony was he died of exposure hanging only ten feet above the ground. Unable to "see" in the dark he was also unable to trust.

Turning again to Webster's Dictionary we find a number of definitions for "trust." The first definition of the <u>noun</u> is **1a:** assured reliance on the character, ability, strength, or truth of someone or something. The first definition of the <u>transitive verb</u> is **1a:** to commit or place in one's care or keeping; **b:** to permit to ... do something without fear or misgiving.

Trust is not something we easily give blindly. This man did not know the character or truth of God. If he had then he would have "cut the rope." He did not know that "God is love" is truth, and that "perfect love casts out fear." If he had, then he would have cut the rope without "fear or misgiving."

We need to know the character and truth of God and this requires diligence and effort. It is in knowing God that we truly have eternal life. John 17:3 says, *"And this is eternal life, that they may know You, the only true God, and Jesus Christ whom You have sent."* Eternal life is not living forever. Eternal life is knowing God and Jesus in fullness. As we come to know them we learn to trust them and we have an "assured reliance on" them and we permit them to operate in our lives "without fear or misgiving."

Discipline is **not** tragedy or calamity. God did not kill this climber but the Bible tells us clearly that the one thing God requires of us is faith. He told the man how to save his life. He even told him the ground was near. The man wanted to "see it" or "feel it" to believe it. Either of those eliminates faith. What we see we don't have to have faith for. God wanted this man to live. God was not mad at him, and God is not mad at you. He is not holding your sins against you. He wants to exchange old for new, and He greatly desires that you become part of His family, through faith in Jesus Christ.

Cut the rope.

Chapter Nine

Bodily Exercise

In ancient times there was not much need for a discussion of exercise. Walking nearly everywhere was commonly accepted practice and even riding was physically challenging enough to generate a calorie burn in the rider. Preparing food required effort as did planting and growing. Only the wealthy were spared many of these activities and even they did not live the life of ease that even many of those below the poverty line experience today.

With television, video games, computers, cars and gadgets galore we have very little reason to exercise but movement and activity are requirements for keeping our body under control. I do not mean that everyone must have an "exercise program," rather that people need movement and activity. If a specific exercise regimen is chosen, fine. If your activity is regular yard work, planting your garden, wrestling with your kids or taking long walks with your spouse don't let it be said that you're failing in your duty to your body as long as you do these things 30 to 45 minutes, at least 3 to 4 days per week.

Paul said, *"For bodily exercise profits a little, but godliness is profitable for all things, having promise of the life that now is and of that which is to come."* (1 Timothy 4:8) There is value in exercise, but that value is minimal compared to the need for godliness.

Before Christ's time Jewish history does not contain many references to games and athletics. The Hebrews took one day off each week to rest, or to keep the Sabbath. The other six days were spent in pursuits, be they financial or spiritual. They were diligent and earnest in business, family and religion.

By the time of Jesus the Hebrew's were under Roman rule. The Romans were greatly influenced by the Grecians in regard to culture and leisure. Games and athletic contests were commonplace throughout the civilized world and Paul grew up exposed to them. He encountered more of these activities as he traveled the known world and many references to soldiering, athletics and farming made their way into his writings. These references once again demonstrate that concept of a "glass darkly" or a "mirror" that we look into. Spiritual things are not exactly like natural analogies but we can use these analogies to help us understand and apply the principles to our lives and gain the desired result.

For example, Paul made specific references to running in 1 Corinthians 9:24-27. In these verses he is comparing the dedication and discipline of runners preparing to race, as well as the participation of all those who enter the race. Some enter a race with insufficient preparation but they are still "in a race" and running along with everyone else. In that running, though, only one brings home the prize.

Even if we consider modern day races in which there are age-group awards, master's awards and often for longer races there are finisher awards, we recognize that in any of those there is only one "winner." From the overall winner to the first in each age group, to the first master runner, one is singled out. This is as it should be. Our human endeavors are enhanced by competition. Without clear winners there is no striving for excellence, no reason for self-discipline; to train hard. Paul said, *"Do you not know that those who run in a race all run, but one receives the prize? Run in such a way that you may obtain it."*

He is admonishing believers to be *"diligent to present yourself approved to God, a worker who does not need to be ashamed, rightly dividing the word of truth."* (2 Ti 2.15) It is easy to be lazy or slothful. It takes no great effort to stay in the house. The book of Proverbs describes the slothful person as one who turns on their bed like a door on its hinges. Diligence, on the other hand, requires commitment and effort.

"And everyone who competes for the prize is temperate in all things." (v. 25a) Temperance is, according to the Webster's

Collegiate Dictionary, Tenth Edition: "Marked by moderation: as **a**: keeping or held within limits: not extreme or excessive: **b**: moderate in indulgence or appetite or desire."

Paul is saying that these athletes lived fasted lifestyles. They did not over-indulge or eat all that they wanted. Those who came out on top lived disciplined lifestyles. After making this point he brings the principle home. *"Now they do it to obtain an imperishable crown, but we for an imperishable crown."* (v. 25b)

He proclaims that in order for us to live victorious lives we too must be "temperate" in all things, at least in all things that relate to the body (see v. 27). We should indulge in reading and studying the word and in spending time with the Lord, but we should not do so in eating, drinking, exercising, television, movies, music, newspapers, books, and etc.

That being said, in verse 27 Paul says, *"I discipline my body and bring it into subjection,"* so that his body won't trip him up as he walks in spiritual things. One method of disciplining our bodies is through exercise. It is not a means of spirituality. Exercise is not vital to our success. There are other means of disciplining the body, specifically prayer and fasting, which should be included in our due diligence regardless of whether we exercise. But exercise does enhance our physical body to the degree that we have a greater energy and mental acuity thus enhancing our lives. And exercise does require discipline.

When people begin to exercise there are a variety of excuses and rationalizations that crop up to allow us to miss our regular exercise. Discipline is required for us to discern these for what they are and to do what we need to in order to exercise. One excuse is, "I just don't feel like it." That is a specific example of the need to discipline the body. Don't ask it how it feels; tell it to get to work.

This concept relates directly to obeying God and also to physical healing. Sometimes we can't "see" why God would tell us to do a certain thing, or we want to believe we're healed but we "feel" sick. Discipline learned through prayer, fasting, exercise and other methods of training your body kicks in. You obey God because you know He's right, regardless of what you see. You cry aloud, "by His stripes I am healed (1 Peter 2:24)" regardless of how you feel, knowing that Jesus has already provided your healing. The louder your senses yell, the more resolute you become because you have already learned to ignore the deception of your senses as you have fasted and prayed and exercised, even when it didn't feel good or seem to make sense.

* * *

I am a runner. My exercise is done on the roads and trails surrounding my community. Running is a fairly simple form of exercise requiring less expensive and exotic equipment than other methods. That doesn't mean it is completely inexpensive. From technical clothing, quality running shoes and race entry fees, there are a number of costs associated with running.

However, there is also a principle of human endeavor. Thomas Paine said it this way, "What we obtain too cheap, we esteem too lightly."

I am a runner. The results I have obtained from running did not come cheap. The monetary expense is only a portion of the cost to which I refer. There has been the cost of rising before the sun on numerous occasions in order to log the requisite miles and still be at work, or to be there for my family. There are the numerous miles I have logged and the time involved in running those miles. There have been bad days and good days, off days and on days. My body has been through the ringer in training and racing.

I have raced 5k to 50 miles. I have completed, at this time, six full marathons (a true marathon is always 26.2 miles in length) including the prestigious Boston Marathon. I finished two ultra marathons, which is any distance longer than the marathon, in 2005. My first ultra was a 50-mile race in northern Michigan and one of the greatest challenges of my life. It was also a tremendous time of revelation.

During the last half of the race I had a revelation of "discipline(ing) my body" and bringing it under subjection. There was a definite point in the race, my wife tells me it was at mile 29.5, in which it would have been very easy to quit, taking the easy way, to listen to my body. I said to her, "This is getting hard." She responded, "Are you going to do this?" She tells me it was a challenge. I didn't recognize that at the moment, but I was challenged inside never the less.

"I'm doing this," I replied, firmly. I grabbed some food and headed back out onto the trail. I'd love to say that it became easier from that moment but it didn't. However, I can say that from that moment there was not another time that I considered quitting. Eventually the race was finished, but the lesson lives on for me.

All of us face challenges in life. Are you going to run your race? Are you going to do this, whatever this is, that God has placed before you? Are you going to listen to your flesh and take the easy way?

Commitment to His word, to His grace will carry you through, but only after you have disciplined your body and brought it under subjection. Fasting specific meals, living a fasted lifestyle, exercise, and prayer; these are all tools that we have to bring our bodies into subjection so that we don't "become disqualified."

For those who have not begun a regular exercise program but wish to there are numerous resources starting with your own local health clubs or running and fitness stores. They can assist you in planning a program that suits your needs and fitness level.

For those who are interested in running there are a few web sites that provide training advice and plans including the web site for the magazine, Runner's World; www.runnersworld.com. There is a good site for those starting out called www.coolrunnings.com.

Many communities have running clubs who love to help new

runners. Many of these can be found on the web with a search for "running clubs."

Contact information for me is provided at the back of the book and I am glad to assist anyone in beginning an exercise program.

Chapter Ten

Building on the Foundation

A recent article in a local periodical stated that most people gain weight as they age. Statistics from a survey said 9 out of 10 women and 7 out of 10 men become overweight as they move into their 40's and beyond. The article seemed to suggest inevitability. Of course it cannot be "inevitable" if it is not 100%.

Even if it is not certain that all will become overweight the numbers suggest that most of us don't stand a chance. Why is it that people become overweight? We understand that for extremely obese people there may be complications that contribute, but in general people become overweight because they eat more calories than their bodies burn.

When we are young our bodies are fat burning machines

provided there is a reasonable degree of activity. It seems that many youths can eat whatever they want and just can't gain weight. However, as you age your metabolism's demands diminish. You reach your full height and you are no longer burning free calories just for growth. If our eating habits do not change at that point we will begin the *almost* inevitable process of becoming overweight.

People do not become overweight by stuffing themselves on Thanksgiving and Christmas. Weight gain is a result of a cumulative practice of eating more calories than we burn. This is not something that happens overnight; rather it is something that compounds over time until we're constantly fighting the battle over our weight.

I graduated from high school at 155 pounds. I graduated from Coast Guard Boot Camp, in Alameda, California, at the same weight just over one year later. I went to my first duty station, USCG Station Muskegon. At that time Station Muskegon was a Search and Rescue (SAR) station. We operated 24 hours a day, 365 days per year. We were split up into duty sections for operations. When I first arrived at the station a duty section had 24-hour duty one day out of three, with one weekend out of three. Our cook prepared meals for breakfast and lunch Monday through Friday with dinner being "open galley" which meant we fended for ourselves. The cook would leave meats and other food items out for the duty section. The entire weekend was "open galley" from Friday dinner. Our first cook would keep lots of treat type items on hand, such as ice cream and soft drinks.

Our work could often be challenging but it was not always particularly active. We stood four-hour radio watches each duty day and again during that night. We sat around and watched television or read much of the time after normal working hours. I arrived at the station in September so we were going into the Great Lakes winter season which meant a significantly reduced case load and far less maintenance work. Our leaders did what they could to keep us busy but we did not train then as Great Lakes units do today, with a significant emphasis on ice rescue. When I was in Muskegon winter was a very sedentary time for a Coastie.

Before we came to spring I had gained 15 pounds. I was stunned when I went to the doctor for some ailment and was told my weight. I had been a runner in high school but I hadn't done much running since basic training. That spring I decided I didn't like what had happened to me and I started running. I lost most of the 15 pounds and kept it off during my Coast Guard years by running, training in the martial arts and running some more.

I was released from Active Duty in the Coast Guard in 1982 but I continued to run. I met my wife a few years later and we're in our 20th year of marriage at this writing. Over the course of these 19+ years my weight gradually crept up to 190-195 pounds. Many people like to blame weight gain on getting married and there is undoubtedly some truth there. We tend to eat more consistently when we're married than when we were single. While we may eat the same number of calories in a meal we often eat fewer meals. If we eat more meals as a married person that will add up to more calories consumed each day. Meanwhile, the demands of marriage, family, work and life tend to reduce our activity levels. This combination often leads to weight creep. Next thing you know, like me, you find yourself 20 or more pounds over what is considered your ideal weight.

Now, remember, your ideal weight is whatever you and God decide it is. There are guidelines in the world which are helpful but I currently weigh 165 pounds at 5'11". The tables say my "ideal" weight is in the neighborhood of 170-175 pounds. I believe that God and I disagree with that. I currently have a body-fat content of between 6-8%. Many ultra runners maintain body-fat at around 5%. Accordingly, I can still lose some fat. That may or may not translate into additional weight lost, depending on whether I add muscle in the process. But someone who is my height and age is considered healthy with a body-fat percent between 17-24%. That could easily translate into an additional 10-15 pounds and that person would be considered "healthy" by most worldly standards.

I have consistently advocated a non-judgmental approach to your weight since the world's view is not God's view. However, there are two caveats or qualifications. First, while God does not look to our outward appearance we must understand that not everything is based on that vertical relationship. That is the context of the book of James. While Romans declares that we are saved, before God, by faith alone, James puts it into practical terms. Our works declare the faith that's in our hearts. In other words, a true salvation experience should produce changes in your heart, thus producing changes in what you do. Being born again is first, but living out your faith, not by duty or require-ment, reveals what took place in your heart by faith.

In the same way people must understand that as a temple of the Holy Spirit we should not allow our bodies to lie in ruin. It is not for you to say, "I know I'm 50 pounds overweight but God is pleased with me so what do I care." It is for you to go before the Lord and seek Him and let Him reveal things to you that need to be changed, including your body composition. He will because He cares. We can "fall short of the Grace of God" (Hebrews 12:15), which means if we abuse ourselves and some-thing bad happens as a result we can't blame God for the result. If we allow ourselves to become, or remain, obese then we can-not say that God is responsible for any attendant health problems.

Second, weight is not the primary measure of health; body composition is. Recall my comments regarding my body fat and so-called healthy body fat for my height. A well-muscled person who is 20 pounds heavier than the average for a person of the same height will most likely have a better body composition, i.e. lower body fat. It is a fact, with regard to this natural world, that fatty tissue that wraps around your organs causes them to have to work harder. As I said, a healthy Body Fat Index (BFI) for the average male is 17-24%. It will not harm you to become acquainted with your BFI.

Remember, though, the most significant measure of health is not your weight but your heart. *"A merry heart does good, like medicine..."* Proverbs 17:22a. One problem with many of the medical studies that are done is that they never take into account the heart, or attitude, of the persons studied. A sad, depressed, pessimistic person is far more likely to contract some disease than one who is filled with love, gratitude or optimism. That could well be the true deciding factor. In fact, I believe the scripture says it is so. In one place we are told, *"the joy of the LORD is your strength."* (Nehemiah 8:10b) and in another it says, *"Keep your heart with all diligence, for out of it spring the issues of life."* (Proverbs 4:23)

Jesus declared that what goes into a man does not defile him, for what goes in is processed and voided through our waste disposal systems. However, that which comes out of our mouths is what defiles us because we speak of adultery, fornication, murder, hate and *"...out of the abundance of the heart the mouth speaks."* (Matthew 15:18-20 and 12:33)

We cannot flaunt our liberty as believers by thinking we can exist solely on ice cream, or even solely on God's word. If we don't practice wise food choices we will reap what we sow in malnutrition, weakness and possibly death. If that happens because of our bad food choices we will not be able to blame God. But our focus should not be on the latest supplement, vitamin, mineral or diet plan. Our focus needs to be on Jesus and His word. As we focus on the Lord, He can direct us through our hearts as to what we should or should not eat. This may be through some nutrition program that already exists or it may be as simple as the government's new food guidelines mentioned early in this book. It may be simpler in that you may eat what you like. Psalm 37:3 tells us to, "Trust in the LORD, and do good;" and we will "feed on His faithfulness." Verse 4 goes on to say, *"Delight yourself also in the LORD, and He shall give you the desires of your heart."*

This verse does not mean that just whatever you want you can have. It does mean that as we are seeking God, as we are making Him our delight and joy in life we will begin to come into unity with Him and the desires of our hearts will be what His desires are for us. Now, there is a definite requirement here. We **must** be delighting ourselves in the Lord. Jesus said it like this in Matthew 6:33 *"Seek first the kingdom of God and His righteousness."*

Let me explain it this way. I do not like yogurt. I don't like the texture or the flavor. Yogurt happens to be one of those foods that nearly every nutrition program says is "Good for you." I don't like it. I've tried to eat it in a smoothie but I didn't like it. The only way I've ever been able to eat it is as a coating on nuts. At least that way the texture is less like itself. Many times I have tried to make myself eat yogurt because it's so "good for you." No go. As I have begun to delight myself in the Lord I have found that I am at peace with not eating yogurt, so I don't. I know that's a small thing, and I know that you can say that can easily be attributed to personal taste. Let me use another food example.

I grew up loving a good steak. My mother and I would buy boxes of frozen steaks so I could have steak two or three times a week. I also liked hamburger. Red meat was good to me. Later in life I made a conscious decision to eat less red meat. Yes, I initially made it because of all the studies. However, as I've learned these truths regarding food choices I have considered having steak on many occasions, particularly when going to dine at a good steakhouse. However, as I've delighted myself in the Lord I have little desire to eat steak. I am not prohibited from it. I do eat the occasional cheeseburger, especially after a 20, or more, mile run. But when I go into that steakhouse I find that I really want that grilled chicken rather than the steak.

I believe that is God leading me in my food choices. I drink Dr. Pepper regularly and enjoy it. My mother thinks I'm killing myself slowly but I have no "desire" to stop drinking it. I do not drink as much as I want to. I do exercise restraint and moderation where Dr. Pepper is concerned, but I do drink it. I am healthy and fit.

Remember, Nehemiah 8:10 starts off, *"Eat the fat, drink the sweet..."* It follows up with *"the joy of the Lord is (our) strength."* Don't allow the world to dictate to you, neither let yourself reject all the guidelines in arrogance. Listen to the Spirit of God in your heart and make wise food choices, remembering that so-called healthier foods are usually less calorie rich. If you eat green beans for example, you can eat an entire can and only consume about 50-60 calories. The same weight of potato chips would be over 400 calories. Four ounces of turkey breast is about 150 calories while the same amount of ice cream is over 600 calories.

Eat the fat, drink the sweet, but remember Paul's instruction to do all natural things in moderation. Moderation is essentially another way of saying a fasted lifestyle. A fasted lifestyle; or moderation, mean simply not eating or drinking all that you want at any time. Meanwhile, we are encouraged to take the word of God to excess. The truths found in God's word are eternal, relevant and life-changing, including these truths we've explored regarding diet, exercise and health. My prayer and hope is that you will be set free from diet-consciousness, but taken in by a God-consciousness and that you will find yourself enjoying food, your family and your life "more abundantly." (John 10:10)

Chapter Eleven

A Plan

Without presenting myself as a dietitian and without trying to put anyone into bondage I am presenting a plan that I have used as I dropped over 25 pounds, including 18 pounds in two months. This isn't my plan, it's a plan I acquired from a magazine and adapted to suit me. The plan in the magazine provided extensive information on foods and the type of nutrients they provide. I will not do that. First, that information is readily available in too many places to cite. Second, that has not been the basis of my success. Remember, this is a plan that worked for me. As I stated earlier, I do not pretend to know what anyone else should eat or what will work best for everyone. You must consider all information carefully and choose for yourself what you believe will work for you.

If you choose to use this plan, or any plan, you must first know two things:

1) In order to lose weight you must burn more calories than you consume.
2) Your current weight.

The plan is based on establishing your base calorie consumption to simply maintain your current weight. In order to do this you multiply your current weight by 10. The next step is to determine how active you are. The chart below will help you determine your level of activity.

Very inactive	(elderly, very low metabolism or very little activity)
Inactive	(an office worker, author or middle-manager)
Slightly inactive	(occasional sports or walking)
Moderately active	(frequent cardio activities)
Highly active	(almost always on the go, seldom sitting or still)
Strenuously active	(High demand physical labor, endurance athlete)

Once you have your base weight x 10 you need to take that number and multiply it by a percentage based on your activity level (see chart on the next page).

Very inactive	20%
Inactive	30%
Slightly inactive	40%
Moderately active	50%
Highly active	60%
Strenuously active	70%

There are two ways to do this and which one you use will determine how conservative you should be with the above categories. The first way, requiring the most conservative choice from above that still allows you enough food for energy and health, is to establish a monthly factor. In other words, today I weigh 166. If I were establishing my calorie consumption for the month I would multiply 166 x 10 which equals 1660. I would then select a category from above. If my goal is to lose weight then I will be conservative without sacrificing health or energy. Although I am an endurance athlete (I average 80 to 100 miles a week) I would choose either "moderately" or "highly active" as opposed to "strenuously active." Let's suppose I select "highly active" for this demonstration. I would then multiply 1660 x .6 and then I would add the result back to 1660.

166 x 10 = 1660 x .6 = 996 + 1660 = 2656

Since I was conservative in my selection I would feel comfortable rounding that total to 2660 for easier use during my daily calorie tracking. 2660 calories would be my allowed consumption every day for the next 30 days. Since my level of activity is normally higher than I allowed for I will be about 150-300 calories under my weight maintenance amount on average (which would be determined by multiplying the higher category percentages by 1660).

It takes about 3500 calories to add or lose one pound. It is also important that I do **not** attempt to get to a 3500 calorie deficit too quickly. If you undercut your calorie intake by more than about 300 calories per day you risk having your metabolism adjust to the larger deficit and begin slowing down. Thus you actually will counteract your weight losses and also put your health at risk. Your body requires sufficient calories to allow all your systems to function at peak. It also requires that you have a balanced intake of carbohydrates (carbs), proteins and fats.

That's right, I said "fats". Of course, as you've no doubt heard, there are "good fats" and "bad fats." In other words, there are some fats that have a greater propensity to assist your body and some that don't. However, again, remember that the key here is a balanced intake. Carbs should make up about 55-60% of your intake, give or take; protein should range between 25-30% and fats should be 10-20%. Those are averages and are not intended to suggest that you "count carbs" or any of the other things. The primary thing is, if you eat a fairly balanced diet, following the basic guidelines provided by the USDA and its Food Pyramid then you will more than likely hit the averages.

By following the above "plan" you would hit that 3500

calorie level every 12-24 days and you should be able to see a pound difference on your scale. There is a caveat. If you have started an exercise program as a part of your new lifestyle then you will be exchanging some fat for muscle. During this process you may not always see weight loss however you should notice some other differences. Your clothes may fit better, or you may see a difference in the mirror while not seeing any on the scale. Lean muscle takes up less space for the same weight than fat. Initially you may see changes in your body composition without seeing large reductions in weight. This is a good thing. Don't be discouraged. Remember, this is a lifestyle change, not a diet. The long-term change is the goal, not the short-term. It's a marathon, not a sprint.

The last item for this option is to point out that you must adjust your calorie level every month. You must use the same scale you previously used, ensure it is calibrated and take your weight under the same or similar conditions that you took it for the first month. I usually take my weight in the morning, prior to my workout. I would need to be sure to do that initially and for each month thereafter. You really do weigh a bit differently depending on the time of day and your level of water weight.

Once I get my new weight, if it is different, I must do the calculations again for the next month. If my weight hasn't changed I will use the same numbers. If my weight hasn't changed at all and I am supposedly averaging 300 calories under per day I would ask a few questions.

First, am I eating breakfast daily? Am I eating high-calorie meals only once or twice per day? Am I eating a high-calorie meal late in the night (or just before I go to bed if I'm an overnight worker)? Have I been honest regarding my serving sizes and calorie counts?

It is important to realize that while your body burns calories like a car burns gasoline you can't store calories like gasoline, in a separate tank. Your body stores extra calories as fat. If you eat a 1250 calorie meal at lunch and another at dinner to make your calorie intake for the day your body will not be able to process all those calories right away. Your body, at rest, burns about 25-50 calories per hour just for breathing and heart beating and thinking and waste processing. What other activity you place on top of that places further demands on your body requiring calories however your body can only process about 250-400 calories per hour. A 1250 calorie meal will supply about 200-400 calories for that hour and the one immediately following. If we say that equals 800 calories your body will not be able to use, immediately, the extra 450 calories. It will convert much of that to fat and store it. Once again, you will be messing up your efforts.

Smaller meals spread over the course of the day produce better results because they better match your body's system design. In addition, eating breakfast is important because you jump start your metabolism after having spent between 6 and 10 hours having it slow down. Just as it is self-defeating to cut calories too quickly, it is also self-defeating to have an unbalanced consumption plan.

I am going to qualify all of the above comments once again.

These are general guidelines and averages. Life sometimes requires us to miss breakfast, or to eat late, or to have a high-calorie meal. Big deal. Go with the flow. The guidelines are provided as a checklist to help you determine what you may be consistently doing that would be sabotaging your efforts.

Of course, the most critical component is being honest regarding your calorie consumption and serving sizes as they relate directly to calorie consumption.

* * *

Well, that takes care of the first option for using this "plan". The second option is similar but is used on a daily basis rather than for a month. Once more you multiply your current weight by 10. You determine your activity level as before, but you must be even more conservative. You are looking at activity other than any exercise you do. Thus I use the "slightly inactive" category based on what I do when I'm not exercising. I sit at my computer, I go to meetings, and on occasion I play actively with my children, other times I sit to play games with them. I multiply the corresponding percent; 40% by 1660. The product is 664 which when I add that to 1660 I get 2324. I have rounded this number to 2300 and I consider that my Base maintenance intake amount for any day that I just do my work without exercise. For all days that I exercise I add the net calories burned to my Base for that day's allowance.

For example, today I ran 6 miles. Based on my Garmin 201 GPS training device I burned 800 calories. From that I subtract the amount I would have burned per hour (which is about 100 calories) if I were not exercising. Although I actually did the run in under an hour (46 minutes) I subtracted 100 calories for ease of use. As a result my allowance for today is 3000 calories. Since I am preparing for a marathon and not trying to lose weight I will attempt to eat all of that 3000 calories, however if I were in a weight loss mode I would try to stay under by about 200 calories.

This second option is the method I have used to drop nearly 30 pounds and keep it off over the past 3 years. I lost 18 pounds in the first two months, 26 pounds in the first six months and I have remained between 164 and 168 for over one year. It does require you to learn to accurately determine portion sizes and to be sure to read labels on products. You need to get a calorie counter book or a chart off the internet and you must get nutrition guides from your favorite restaurants. Yes, darn it, there is some "work" to do. But diligence in this arena, as with any other, will produce the desired results. Proverbs 12:24 says, *"The hand of the diligent will rule, but the lazy man will be put to forced labor."* Proverbs 10:4 says, *"He who has a slack hand becomes poor, but the hand of the diligent makes rich."*

The principle found in these two verses applies to life in general and to the responsibility we have over our bodies. I desire that you enjoy life and food and I believe we are free from laws governing our food choices. We are not free from taking responsibility for our bodies as the temple of the Holy Spirit.

Chapter Twelve

Biblical Healing

Many diet, nutrition and exercise books are written to suggest that these are the means to better health. If you eat certain foods, take in certain nutrients or perform certain exercises you will build a healthier, happier you. Millions of people buy into the message every year and some even get the results they're looking for; a firmer mid-section, reduced thighs, pumped up chest or even more energy and vitality as advertised.

There are testimonials of numerous people beating cancer through one diet method or another. There are stories of people who were caught in the midst of depression but ran their way out. The anecdotal information supports all the claims made by all the purveyors of change that will be brought about by following their method.

Meanwhile, for every story of success there are at least two stories of failure. For every person who loses that extra 50 pounds there are many more out there who just can't do it. They fight with themselves, they battle against the images our society promotes and they lose. For some the loss is of life, as they fight with one disease or another.

I would like to tell you that the truths I've shared would keep anyone who applied them from dying but that would be misleading. Often we battle years and years of programming and we just come to the fight with new weapons too late. A person who is diagnosed with cancer does not stand a chance if they are predisposed to believing that cancer is a death sentence. All the new weapons available will not help them at all if they do not believe.

I say this in relation to nearly every testimony of success available, whether it came through diet, nutrition, exercise, medicine or God's power alone. Jesus made a declaration in Matthew 9:29. *"According to your faith let it be to you."* To the woman with the issue of blood he said, *"Daughter, be of good cheer, your faith has made you well."* (Matthew 9:22)

In Mark 10:51 Jesus ministered to a blind man. The man said, "I want to see," and Jesus replied, *"Go your way, your faith has made you well,"* and in Luke 17, Jesus told the leper, *"Your faith has made you well."*

The lesson in these verses is clear; we receive from God according to what we believe from God. Now, before you finally toss this book out and label me a heretic, let me qualify the above. I do not believe that it is <u>faith</u> alone that gets God to move, or to provide some thing for us. However, Hebrews 11 makes it very clear that it is <u>faith</u> alone that pleases God. And the above cited verses make it very clear that the faith of these people had to be in operation to receive healing. Their faith, any faith, does not **have power**. Faith is what **receives** power. The power is, was, and always shall be God's power. I do not force God to release His power with my faith. These people did not force Jesus to heal them; He was already predisposed to release God's power in their lives. We see that truth revealed in Acts 10:38; *"how God anointed Jesus of Nazareth with the Holy Spirit and with power, who went about <u>doing good and healing all</u> who were oppressed by the devil, for God was with Him."*

Jesus never met a person He didn't want to heal. If you read the Gospels you will find that Jesus was constantly described as healing <u>all</u> their sick folk. In the above verse it states that He *"went about ... healing all who were oppressed by the devil."* What it doesn't say is that He ever went anywhere and put any sickness on anybody. Does it? It says He healed those who were "oppressed by the devil." Now, Hebrews 1 tells us Jesus was the express image of God, or the exact representation of the Father. This verse in Acts 10 tells us Jesus was doing these things because "God was with Him." If Jesus never put any sickness on anyone while He walked the earth then what makes people think God is doing that today?

The only people Jesus didn't heal in large numbers were people in Nazareth, his hometown. The Gospels describe the reason. In Nazareth the people were so familiar with the man,

Jesus-bar-Joseph, that they could not accept Him as anything but a human. (Matthew 13:54-58, Mark 6:1-6) They did not operate in faith, which would have allowed them to look beyond the natural man that grew up there. *"Now He could do no mighty work there, except that He laid His hands on a few sick people and healed them. ⁶And He marveled because of their unbelief."* (Mark 6:5-6a)

There are only two places recorded in the Gospels that say Jesus "marveled." One was here in Mark 6 and the other was in relation to the Roman centurion's faith. (Matthew 8:5-13; Luke 7:1-10) This centurion did not require that Jesus come to his house and do some mystical thing, only that He would speak the word "and my servant will be healed." The centurion explained his understanding of authority and Jesus was amazed at the centurion's "great faith."

Faith can be described as a confidence in the word, character or integrity of another. God's word plainly declares that Jesus came to heal us. (More on this later.) His word also states that it is impossible for God to lie; He has great integrity. Jesus came and demonstrated God's character of Love by the way He lived, and the way He died. God is someone we can have <u>faith</u> in.

Recall that I said that people will not be helped "if they do not believe." I have described above how that applied to the ministry of Jesus, and by extension, to us in receiving from God. It also applies, in principle, to many things in this world. If we don't believe in something, it is most likely that we will not reap any, or at least only limited, benefits from that something.

If a person does not believe that the medicine the doctor is offering them will help, then most likely that medicine will not help. If you don't believe in the nutrition plan or exercise plan you are about to embark on, then most likely you will not stay with it long and you will not reap any benefits from it. As Paul said, if you believe you can only eat vegetables, then you should only eat vegetables.

The good news is we can change what we believe. In this natural world we can listen to the doctor and rehearse their words; we can read stories of how the medicine helped others and imagine this medicine helping us. We can talk to ourselves about the wonders of medical science and about how we are not ready to give up. As we do these things our minds will begin to see a different outcome.

While these methods have not always produced the desired result if you read the stories of success you will see that each of them could "see" success inside before they experienced it in their lives or bodies.

I am not advocating any kind of mysticism or "imaging" techniques. I am merely stating that people already receive "according to" their faith, and that faith, or what we believe, can be changed as we listen to instruction and see the principles working for us.

These are biblical principles and they are universal in that God put these principles into operation in the earth and because it was God, they work. Now, these principles have only limited success without being empowered by the Holy Spirit in our lives.

And these principles often only have limited success even when we are looking to God's word because we struggle with our own inability to believe what God has promised us. We look at how we feel, and what our situation is, and we believe that is the truth. Jesus said, *"I am the way, the truth, and the life."* (John 14:6) In John chapter One and in 1 John chapter One the scripture reveals that Jesus is the Living Word.

The things that are written are expressions of God's nature and character. In Matthew 8, we find Jesus casting out devils and healing all that were sick once again (v. 16). In verse 17 Matthew explains why, *"that it might be fulfilled which was spoken by Isaiah the prophet, saying: He Himself took our <u>infirmities</u> and bore our <u>sicknesses</u>."* This is a quote from Isaiah 53:4, except that Isaiah used two different words.

> ⁴Surely He has borne our <u>griefs</u> and carried our
> <u>sorrows</u>; Yet we esteemed Him stricken, smitten
> by God, and afflicted.

The use of "infirmities" and "sicknesses" by Matthew, under the inspiration of the Holy Spirit, makes it clear that the statement in the verse below, "by His stripes we are healed," is referring to physical healing for our bodies.

> ⁵But He *was* wounded for our transgressions, *He
> was* bruised for our iniquities; the chastisement
> for our peace *was* upon Him, and by His stripes
> we are healed.

The Greek word most often translated "saved" is *sodzo* and

is often translated "made whole" in reference to physical healing (Matthew 9:22; Mark 5:34; Luke 8:48). There are a number of scriptures that join our physical healing to the forgiveness of sins (Psalms 103:3; Isaiah 53:4-6; and 1 Peter 2:24). Healing is just as much a part of our salvation as forgiveness.

If you don't believe this, you will not experience it. You will receive from God only that which you believe for from God. It is not only as simple as a lack of faith that prevents receiving, but it is certain that if you do lack faith you will not receive.

I say again, healing is *from* God. It is received by faith, but it is a gift of God's Grace. If it were not apportioned to us in the work that Jesus did on the cross no amount of "believing" would make it so.

In this chapter I have described the relationship of faith to receiving any benefits in life. While faith in natural things is not comparable to faith in God, the principle is. The bottom line for you, to use that tired cliché, is; **what are you going to believe?**

Are you going to put your faith in pills, diets and nutrition plans and find yourself in bondage to a lifestyle that may or may not give you relief in this life? Or, are you going to put your faith in God and His word, and find yourself liberated from all the "rules" of dieting and enjoy freedom in this life **and** realize eternal benefits?

The choice is yours, choose wisely.

For an excellent teaching on biblical healing I strongly recommend, "God Wants You Well" from Andrew Wommack

Ministries. He has a tape series and a booklet with the same title. In addition to the website already given you can write to his ministry at:

P.O Box 3333
Colorado Springs, CO 80934-3333
You can call them at 719-635-1111.

Chapter Thirteen

Finally!

God is a good God. He wants you well. He desires that you have a happy and blessed life. He gives you all those things so that you can give them away.

Seriously, God wants you to share what you have. In Matthew 10 Jesus told His disciples to go out and preach that the kingdom of heaven was at hand, which meant it was being demonstrated to them right now. In verse 8 he added these instructions: *"Heal the sick, cleanse the leper, raise the dead, cast out devils. Freely **you have received, freely give."** He didn't give them power and anointing just for them; He gave it so they could share it. Our lives would be full and rich and filled with purpose if we would simply live them committed to this truth, "freely you have received; freely give."

The great and glorious God gives to you in abundance so you may give to others, but He always gives more than we can imagine if we'll let Him. He does this to make sure we have enough, too. Focus on the giving, not the getting. Don't apply the principles in this book merely for your gain (or loss, of weight, that is). Apply the principles so you will be at your best and in your best health so that you can be a living epistle "known and read by all men." (2 Co 3:2) Let God's life and love show so that others will be challenged to know Him.

God bless you in all your days as you live joyously for Him.

A New Life

While many of the principles found in this book can be used by anyone, the strength of these truths is found in living the "born again" life. In John 3:3 Jesus told Nicodemus, a ruler of the Jews, *"Most assuredly, I say to you, unless one is born again, he cannot see the kingdom of God."*

Nicodemus didn't understand so Jesus explained that it is being born of the Spirit, not the flesh. Everyone experienced the birth of the flesh in this world. Jesus said that a new birth, a birth of the Spirit, is required to go to heaven **and** to experience all the benefits of grace in this life.

If you have never made Jesus Lord of your life as Romans 10:9-10 says; *"that if you confess with your mouth the Lord Jesus and believe in your heart that God has raised Him from the dead, you will be saved. For with the heart one believes unto right-eousness, and with the mouth confession is made unto salvation (born again, new birth)"*; you can do so right now. You can accept Jesus this moment. I know faith has been initiated in your heart as you've read this book. Your heart is stirred to action; don't "fall short of the grace of God." Pray this prayer:

"Father, I believe that Jesus was raised from the dead, that He has cleansed all my sins. I call Jesus Lord of my life right now and according to your word I believe You have saved me. I give thanks for all that Jesus did and I thank you for giving me a new life right now, in Jesus name, Amen."

If you prayed that prayer please contact us and let us know so we may rejoice with you and provide resources to help you grow in your new life.

About the Author

Drew Williams is Founder and Pastor of The Harbor. The church is officially known as The Harbor Church of Grand Blanc, Inc., and began its history as Light Fellowship Church in 1997.

Pastor Drew is a competitive runner at many distances and has completed several marathons and two ultramarathons. His wife of 20 years works with him in the church. Mary supports his racing and recently completed her first 10-mile race in August of 2005. She braved rain and humidity to finish her longest race ever, making Drew proud!

Pastor Drew and Mary desire to see you live healthy all the time and are interested in helping you understand God's way to victory. You may contact them through the church:

The Harbor Church
P.O. Box 156
Grand Blanc, MI 48480
810-606-0292
theharborgb@sbcglobal.net

#   #   #